the
hip chick's
guide to
macrobiotics

the hip chick's guide to macrobiotics

a philosophy for achieving a radiant mind and fabulous body

JESSICA PORTER

AVERY

A MEMBER OF PENGUIN GROUP (USA) INC. | NEW YORK

Most Avery books are available at special quantity discounts for bulk purchase for sales promotions, premiums, fund-raising, and educational needs. Special books or book excerpts also can be created to fit specific needs. For details, write Penguin Group (USA) Inc. Special Markets, 375 Hudson Street, New York, NY 10014.

a member of
Penguin Group (USA) Inc.
375 Hudson Street
New York, NY 10014
www.penguin.com

Library of Congress Cataloging-in-Publication Data

Porter, Jessica.
The hip chick's guide to macrobiotics : a philosophy for achieving a radiant mind and fabulous body /
Jessica Porter.
p.   cm.
Includes bibliographical references and index.
ISBN 1-58333-205-7
1. Macrobiotic diet—Recipes.   I. Title.
RM235.P67 2004   2004046273
613.2'5—dc22

Printed in the United States of America
16 18 20 17 15

Book design by Stephanie Huntwork

ACKNOWLEDGMENTS

First of all, this book would basically stink up your kitchen without the patience and generosity of Lisa Silverman and Dr. Marc Van Cauwenberghe. You are true friends, and I owe you both many dinners at Fore Street.

I WOULD ALSO LIKE TO GIVE MASSIVE THANKS TO:

Michio and the late Aveline Kushi, without whose work this book could not have been written.

My mother, Susan McCutcheon, for letting me splash around inside her, and for being a lovely, lovely person.

My father, Julian Porter, for his love, enthusiasm, and performer's genes.

My stepfather, Bob, for his horrible puns, open heart, and big spirit.

My stepmother, Anna, for her priceless diamonds of encouragement.

My sisters, Sue, Cath, and Juls, for each being so amazing in her own way.

Janet Ozzard for being such a close friend and giving endless hours of feedback.

Amy Jenkins for her cool English accent, refreshing honesty, and solid friendship.

Howard for being Howard and living the big life.

Michael, Doug, Aimee, and Keith for exercising my heart during the writing of this book.

William Spear for being so deep, so real, and so funny.

My agent, Diane Gedymin, for "digging" the whole thing when others didn't.

My editor, Kristen Jennings, for her kind and watchful eye.

Gwyneth Paltrow and Madonna for making me see that this stuff is cooler than I thought.

Mick Jagger for getting me through adolescence.

Adam Bock for his Canuck sensibility.

Simon Doonan and Jonathan Adler for supporting this wacky chick.

Susan Trabucchi for laughing out loud.

Marc Gup for kicking my butt.

Kimberly McCall for being my marketing angel.

Kimberly Mngqibisa for being an actual angel.

Lyn Lutrzykowski for her loving help and gentle prodding.

Jane Quincannon for making it all seem so easy.

Gerry Kein, my hypnosis teacher, who taught me all about confidence.

OTHERS WHO MIDWIFED THIS PROJECT:

A deep appreciation goes to Mona Panici for being the first person I shared this project with and who treated it with such tender care. Also to Lynne Rowe, Jon Radtke, Louis Fredrick, Kent Pierce, Pete Leja, Ned Menoyo, Kirstin Millikin, Jenny Coose, Chris Coose, Amy Rolnick, Meg Wolff, Lance Cromwell, Danielle Gorman, Sheila Jackson, Richard Mullen, Sandra Manesky, and anyone else who encouraged me while I birthed this sucker.

SPECIAL THANKS TO MY MACRO TEACHERS:

Lino Stanchich, Christina Pirello, Carry Wolf, Denny Waxman, Michelle Nemer, Joshua Rosenthal, John Kozinski, the Eskos, Diane Avoli, Mary Creighton, Harriet McNear, Blake Gould, Murray Snyder, Bill Tara, Miria Pencke, and all the others who brought their whole selves to this work.

LEST I FORGET:

The Infinite Universe & Bill W.

CONTENTS

Foreword   *ix*

Preface   *xi*

Introduction   *1*

PART ONE
life lessons: the 12 laws of change of the infinite universe

1. Laws 1, 2, and 3   *15*
   Snack Break   *28*

2. Laws 4 and 5   *32*
   McHeartbreak   *38*

3. Laws 6, 7, 8, and 9   *44*
   Rice Break   *51*

4. Laws 10, 11, and 12   *58*

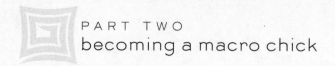

PART TWO
becoming a macro chick

5. Phase One: Going with the Grain   71

6. Phase Two: Cupboard Conversion   95

7. Phase Three: Going Whole Hog   147

8. More Recipes   184

9. Beyond the Diet: Desludging and the Yin and Yang of Love   242

    Conclusion   274

Glossary of Terms   276

Bibliography   280

Resources   282

Index   285

In 1978, my wife Aveline and I founded the Kushi Institute to teach, guide, and motivate individuals to greater personal freedom, health, and happiness through macrobiotics. Inspired by many thinkers and philosophers, including George Ohsawa, we came to appreciate the importance of food as our biological, biopsychological, and biospiritual foundation. The institute is now the leading macrobiotic center in the world and hosts teaching seminars, retreats, training classes, and special programs for health recovery.

It inspires me to see a new generation coming to macrobiotics who are young, vital, and in good health—people who want to live their lives more fully and naturally. It is these people who, by practicing macrobiotics in their daily lives, can go on to fulfill their dreams and live truly great (macro) lives (bios). And their actions are global: when many people are healthy and happy, and live in harmony with nature, the world becomes a more peaceful place. These days, we need macrobiotic foods and principles more than ever.

I have known Jessica Porter for more than ten years; she is a performer, a teacher, and a very funny lady. Because of her playful spirit, she has the ability to communicate macrobiotic ideas to those who learn through laughter. I trust you will enjoy this book, and I wish you congratulations as you embark on your wonderful macrobiotic adventure.

Michio Kushi
Becket, Massachusetts

We all bitch and moan about freedom. And it's important. If you live in North America, chances are you are free from overt oppression. You could even be free of economic want. It is your inalienable right to choose your religion, your shoes, and your cat. It is still possible to walk down the street without being microchipped, and you're free to eat at McDonald's any day of the week. All these freedoms are important and real.

But are you free within your own body? Or do you struggle against yourself, mentally and emotionally? Do you feel a connection to nature? To whatever you call "God"? Are you free of medication? Do you experience your creativity in joyous ways? Are you uninhibited in your sex life? Do you feel good about your relationships? Are you ridiculously happy?

Me neither. But I'm better than I used to be.

These freedoms are easily as important as the political and social ones, but we cannot achieve them through legislation. Fortunately, and unfortunately, it is each person's responsibility to discover and explore those deep, inner freedoms. For some, that comes through organized religion, for others it may be going to the gym. Still others, not knowing how to pursue these invisible goals, shut down, turn on the TV, and ignore their inner worlds completely.

This book is about freedom and food. I believe that what you put in your mouth has a direct impact on your freedom—physically, emotionally, mentally, and spiritually. We can eat in ways that repress our life force, making us into passive automatons within our culture. Or we can eat to be free, connected, and responding to the larger natural world that created us, and continues to create us. The more we eat natural foods and understand the laws of the universe, the more our spirits play freely within it.

Freedom is not chaos. It is not the right or ability to simply do whatever I want whenever I want. True freedom depends upon discovering one's own personal inner compass and following its direction. This occurs in a healthy body that understands and respects the Order of the Universe, laws that the Western world has yet to consciously embrace. When the simple rules of yin and yang are respected, freedom follows naturally.

These laws are exquisitely democratic, and all violations of the laws produce consequences, no matter who you are; the millionaire in the limo has a colon that's rusting out. I can complain all I want, but sugar still gives me cavities. "The president will see you now," but only if his prostate hasn't exploded. Even celebs like Madonna and Gwyneth Paltrow—recent macro devotees—are happier when they eat healthy food. Even *they* must look inside themselves and on their dinner plates for true freedom. Yin and yang rule the day.

The world can only change through the humans that inhabit it. When we as individuals are free and healthy, we tend to affect our families in a positive way; our communities benefit, too. We can legislate all we want, trying to pin our souls' happiness to the ground with laws and statutes. But until we go inside, discovering and responding to our own inner compass, we become miserable trying to create a false freedom on the outside.

The Hip Chick's Guide to Macrobiotics is about ideas as much as it is about food. Take in the philosophy at your own pace. I found that I needed to eat whole foods for a while before the big ideas really started to sink in. If you've already been dabbling in Eastern thought, you may dive straight into yin and yang very easily. I have inserted funny little stories within the philosophy to give your mind a break from all the thinking. But whatever you do, don't ignore the philosophy completely. It is very important in helping to keep you inspired and to fuel your inner freedom.

Please keep studying macrobiotics. Buy other people's books. Get a personal consultation. Go to cooking classes, dinner lectures, or start a potluck. Yin and yang will keep you interested and awake for a lifetime, and there is no end to what they can teach all of us. Meet others who practice macrobiotics. Seek out those with gleams in their eyes, and senses of humor, and learn from them. If you need help from a therapist or a support group to move through heavy feelings or issues, by all means seek it out. I certainly did. But always remember that your intuition, as it is strengthened with macrobiotic food, will eventually become your ultimate authority.

Finally, I hope you make friends with this book, referring to it and rereading it whenever necessary. May it feed you, inspire you, and make you laugh till the carrot juice spews out your nose.

Sincerely,
Jessica Porter

M ore than a diet, macrobiotics is a philosophy. "Macro" means large and "bio" means life. It is the art of creating a big life—a rich, full, exciting life. But how? It is by tuning into how the universe functions that we live the big life. This begins by understanding the grand forces that govern us—basically, the pulse of the universe. The universe expands, and the universe contracts. Whether you call it "God," "Goddess," "Great Spirit," or "Hey, You!" we are all products of this active, pulsing creation; our hearts beat, our lungs fill and empty, our pupils dilate and contract. As we learn the steps of this dance, we become more graceful, happy, and free.

the diet

The Standard Macrobiotic Diet is a template that was created by Michio Kushi, a student of George Ohsawa's, for a presentation he made to the U.S. Congress in the 1970s. They are sound recommendations for developing a sense of balance and strengthening one's health. I mention it here because it is the most recognized set of macrobiotic guidelines that exists. The foods included in the Standard Diet are whole grains, a variety of vegetables, beans and bean products, sea vegetables, soups, pickles, desserts, condiments, and nonaromatic teas. Occasional foods include fish, fruit, and some alcoholic beverages. Normally eschewed are highly refined sugars, chemicalized and processed foods, nightshade vegetables, dairy products, eggs, and most other animal foods (except fish).

However, nothing is forbidden in the practice of macrobiotics because more than anything, macrobiotics is about freedom—the freedom you enjoy as an inhabitant of the universe. You are free to make your choices, and you are free to feel the consequences. It is only through testing the limits of the physical world that we recognize and harmonize with the principles that govern it. Some people need to get an expensive ticket before learning to drive at a moderate speed, just as you may need to feel the headache of a Twinkie binge to truly appreciate brown rice. You are a growing, learning, organic work in progress, and you are free to learn the principles of the universe your way—through pain or through pleasure—on your own timetable. Once the inner compass is discovered and relied upon, all limitations become obsolete.

Also, the macrobiotic diet is different for everyone; kids and parents have different needs, as do men and women. A lumberjack will crave a dinner altogether inappropriate to a monk. It's just a matter of what your goals are. If you want to feel peaceful and connected to nature, you may choose to let go of processed, chemicalized, refined foods. If you are interested in healing your body, you may adopt the standard macrobiotic diet for a while. If you are a boxer, you may want to eat more animal food for physical strength. Whatever brings you closer to your dream in life is what is right for you. And for most people who practice macrobiotics over the long haul, there are vicissitudes. And yes, binges. Whether it's on ice cream or just too many almond butter balls, macrobiotic people, like everyone else, have their own strange food peccadilloes. But when the macrobiotic person makes the journey back to "normal," it is to the peaceful, soft, and forgiving bed of whole grains and other natural foods.

gain grain

The principal food in macrobiotic practice is whole grain. Not whole-grain bread, or whole-grain noodles (although they are eaten as well), but whole grains. The actual little grains themselves—intact. This "wholeness" is essential not only to physical health but also to mental stability and spiritual connectedness. The energy packed into a little whole grain is so strong that, left in its hull, undisturbed, it will endure for centuries, even millennia. Although the recent carbophobia that has swept the nation has finally brought to our consciousness the deleterious effects of refined and processed sugars, we have yet to shine our cultural spotlight on the lowly, yet noble, whole grain.

If you are in good health, you don't have to make any radical changes. Too many times, I have been hired by people to "make them macrobiotic." The first day of the job was spent going through the cupboards like a SWAT team, letting fly crackers, candies, and Coke. By the end of the day, the client was left with some austere glass jars full of ugly dried seaweed and the quivering lower lip of a five-year-old. All this book asks you to do, at first, is GAIN GRAIN in your life. Allow grain to work its wonderful voodoo on you, and your journey will unfold the way it is supposed to. If you are turned on by the changes that occur, you can move on to phases two and three—YOU may be the one throwing out the candies eventually.

the benefits

By practicing macrobiotics, you will achieve a radiant mind because eating whole grains produces a more holistic way of thinking. It makes sense that eating foods created by nature helps us to harmonize with natural rhythms, while eating foods made in a factory helps us to harmonize with video games. By tuning in to the bigger forces, we are freed from former limits; illnesses reverse themselves, unnecessary conflicts disappear, and we become peaceful, playful, and free. Reflecting more deeply, we discover that our biggest problems are actually our teachers, and we end up tipping our hats to our enemies for helping us grow.

Practicing macrobiotics will also lead to a balanced, healthy physical life, but remember: weigh your soul, not your body. My weight has stayed the same for the last seven years as I hit my mid-thirties, and I rarely think about it. It is very rare for macrobiotic people to be overweight. Wholesome foods actually nourish the body, as opposed to starving it, creating beautiful skin, shiny hair, smooth energy. As the body feels happy and nourished, it lets go of excess, dropping it like luggage in the lobby of the Plaza. In our quest to serve the mental images of perfection we carry around, we are tragically starving ourselves of the actual

george

This whole thing began when a Japanese boy watched his two little sisters die of tuberculosis. And then his mother. And then his brother. A scourge in Japan at the time, "consumption" was having its way with this island population. At fifteen, Yukikazu Sakurazawa himself came down with the disease, probably coughing blood into a hankie, as most of our great consumptive protagonists do, and knew he was going to die. But instead of playing endless Nintendo, or visiting a geisha, or any other thing that your average teenage boy might do upon hearing the death knell, Yukikazu decided to fight back.

Yukikazu's mother, having studied Western nutrition, fed her children lots of eggs and dairy food, and, in 1912, Japanese cuisine was thoroughly awash in polished grains. The vital integrity of the whole grain of rice, the staple of this exceptionally strong nation until recent times, had been lost. Like truffles or caviar for us, white rice had become the "cool" thing to eat, as it was considered classy and nutritionally superior. Luckily, there was a doctor at the time, Sagen Ishizuka, treating very ill patients with natural food. Dr. Ishizuka believed that everyone was falling ill precisely because stripping the grain had skewed the natural sodium/potassium balance of the food and, as a result, had left the people stripped of their natural balance as well. Yukikazu heard about this doctor and, with the desperation of a dying man, jumped on the bandwagon.

At nineteen years old, he returned to brown rice. And vegetables. A little oil and some sea salt. He eschewed the sugar, eggs, and dairy products that had crept their way into society and his body. Day by day, little by little, Yukikazu restored his health and his strength. After a few months, the TB was completely cured. Not only had this boy come out the other side of disaster a man of glowing health, he had opened spiritually, too; the energy that had pushed his healing, what he would call the "Infinite Universe," urged him to spread the news of this natural cure to the entire world. Freedom and enthusiasm exploded from his every pore. He had seen the light, and it was on his plate.

George was a cowboy with a genuine lust for true freedom. He believed that life is to be lived as freely and as playfully as possible. Ohsawa even treated his body like a chemistry set, inviting illnesses upon himself in order to cure them. Before he died, he was working on a health-food root beer made from several herbs as a macrobiotic treat.

George Ohsawa distilled the universe into some tidy theorems. Among them, the "Twelve Laws of Change"* are my favorites. He laughed and lectured and served brown rice, insisting that world peace would begin in the body of the individual through biological health. Ohsawa knew from his own experience that we could turn suffering into happiness very easily by eating whole foods and embracing the order of the universe. A voracious reader, constantly tackling the works of the greatest minds of both Western and Eastern cultures, George found in every great tome, every enduring philosophy, even in the Bible, the simple laws of yin and yang.

───────────

*In this book, I have used a combination of George's exact wording of the laws and some rewording that was done by Michio Kushi, currently the most prolific and well-known macrobiotic teacher in the world.

nourishment—physical, emotional, and spiritual—we can derive from healthy food. Feed it well, and your exquisite body will reveal itself to you.

Macrobiotics is not just about food. In this book you will study what are called the Twelve Laws of Change of the Infinite Universe, all of which help us to see how the basic forces of the universe work. It is by aligning with the universe, or "God," that we feel peace and happiness; we can hook up with this power through prayer, meditation, fellowship, and service. In macrobiotics, it is understood that the more we eat natural, energized foods, the more we can sense our intuition, which is our direct line to the universe. In this book, I have created exercises to strengthen your "inner compass" and help you sense your relationship to the bigger picture.

You don't have to follow the diet flawlessly in order to experience the benefits; I certainly don't. While your diet may never be perfect, your relationship to the universe can feel perfectly satisfying every moment. And happily, the more you hook up with the Infinite Universe in your way, the more your body will actually gravitate toward whole foods. I used to practice macrobiotics very rigidly—beating myself up whenever I ate junky foods—because I was afraid of wrecking my chances at "perfect" health. But I had to remember that no one is gettin' out of here alive. This is not about immortality, or perfection, or escap-

for readers with serious health concerns

For Readers Facing Serious Health Challenges: if you are being challenged by a serious illness, this book should serve only as a primer for you. It would be helpful for you to find a qualified macrobiotic counselor (see Resources, p. 282) and get specific dietary recommendations to balance your condition. You will not find them in this book. This book was *not* written to reverse specific physical illnesses. Let this book inspire you, be a teacher to your loved ones, and keep you spiritually engaged. I suggest you read the stories of others who have recovered and surround yourself with loving, positive people looking to achieve the same goals. Fear not: in many ways, you are the luckiest of readers because you are taking a crash course on the secrets of the universe. It is possible to experience amazing, breathtaking changes. I have met hundreds of people like you, who have made it through their odysseys completely transformed and profoundly happy.

Pregnant? If you're pregnant, or even think you may be, check with your caregiver before making any radical changes in your eating, and follow his/her advice. Although adding whole grains to your diet is good for you (and your baby), going on a strict desludging diet is *not* appropriate for making babies. Pregnancy is a time of building, and a strict macro diet is about releasing excess. Macrobiotic women tend to loosen up their diets, obeying their natural cravings during pregnancy.

ing the challenges of being human. Instead, it's about diving deep into this mysterious gift called life. Macrobiotic practice has helped me to enjoy my freaky journey from a free and flexible consciousness; I take no medications, my energy is young and vital, and my relationships feel smooth, honest, and loving. I get to experience my creativity every day, and I am of service to other people. I used to treat macrobiotic practice as an insurance policy against illness, but there is no such thing. Instead, I see it now as a rock-solid investment in a full and rich life. We all die—that is a given. But do we all truly live?

my sludge

In my household growing up, cooking consisted of opening cans and heating up the contents. Dessert was diet ice cream straight from the freezer, and TV dinners were culinary touchdowns. During my glorious high-school years, I worshiped at the altar of the microwave.

It's not that my mother wasn't a good cook; in fact, when she had to impress guests, she could produce the most fantastic roast beef, complete with her mind-blowing gravy and yummy potatoes, topped off with a shiny cherry cheesecake. She just didn't enjoy cooking. And I understand that. Cooking can be a drag.

So it wasn't until I had my own apartment during junior year of college that I was confronted with the challenge of cooking for myself. It was crazy that I had studied five foreign languages, some basic psychoanalytic theory, and dabbled in geology before I ever contributed consciously to what went in my mouth.

Of course, I started with noodles. Who doesn't? My first gourmet exploits consisted of making a huge plate of Ronzoni spaghetti, covered in a bottle of Ragu, my personal touch being the half can of Kraft Parmesan cheese melted in during the heating of the sauce. Of course this daily fare produced fabulous results: pudginess, sloth, and a wonderful lack of direction. And luckily, after a couple of years, I knew I needed a change.

I stood in my kitchen, hands on hips, apron over belly, pushing the ancestral envelope beyond my mother's distaste for cooking. Oh, to be the noble spearhead of humankind's evolution! In that very moment, the universe demanded that I learn how to cook—actual food.

But where would I start? I didn't even know what qualified as real food. Did this mean . . . vegetables? Did this mean cleaning things and (oh, God) cutting things? I became frightened and exhausted just thinking about it. No way. I didn't have the time. I didn't have the . . . ROOM! Surely vegetables took up too much space, with all their leaves and dirt and roots. There was absolutely no way. Not in my tiny New York apartment!

To really, really cook, I needed a sumptuous, sprawling mansion complete with pantry and root cellar somewhere in Connecticut abutting a country club golf course! I needed perfect sunny days and angelic blond children laughing softly around my ankles. I needed nothing less than a six-burner stove with copper-bottom pans and a vast expanse of cutting boards to do justice to my Iron Chef techniques. Everybody knows that dinky Manhattan kitchens can accommodate a toaster and a coffeemaker and that's it. It was painfully obvious: I was a victim of circumstance, and I simply couldn't do it. Too bad.

God bless Ben and Jerry. Two simple moves: open freezer, dip spoon. Nice and easy. I luxuriated for a while in my cool, chocolatey lunch, letting my thoughts roam like a junkie. I would probably have to read a book, right? No, no. Take a class. But wait. Were there actual cooking classes? The question cocked my head. For a split second, I honestly wasn't sure. It seemed like something out of a Stanley Kubrick movie: a person demonstrating to other humans how to manipulate and handle food over fire struck me as so strange—both futuristic and caveman-ish—that I couldn't fit it in my head. A cooking class? Did people actually do that? And then I remembered that my sister had taken a cooking class once. Back in high school she had a big crush on a macrobiotic guy. For a whole summer she got into it, buying books and going to freaky restaurants. I wondered if it was really worth it . . . the guy was very cute.

Cut to: rice. Brown rice. The teacher washes it by swirling it around in water and pouring the water off. Then she does it again. And now she's measuring the water, which is the actual water it's gonna cook in. Pouring it in, carefully, so as not to "disturb the energy of the rice." Excuse me? Come again? Disturb the . . . what? I squelch my perverse urge to interject: "Better be quiet! I wouldn't want to WAKE UP THE RICE!" Ha ha ha. I am killing myself inside. These people are whacked. Get a grip. Get a *life!*

The class is dull, dull, dull. No loud and flamboyant Italian chef sprinkling "essence" over every dish, no funny Martin Yan, not even a George Foreman grill being hawked. Just a woman, who looks exceedingly . . . human. Like an anatomical doll complete with smooth, shiny skin and veins protruding in exactly the right places, she has an almost creepy consistency to all her bits and pieces. For instance, the skin of my thighs can look pretty different from that of my hands, or my chest, or my face. On any given day, my two hands can seem different, one blotchy, the other smooth. But she looked like she had been sewn together with just one piece of skin, everything harmonious, together, complete, like a football. She emitted a translucence that was far from unattractive but dangerously close to unnerving. The whites of her eyes too white, too . . . alive.

I wasn't sure about this whole thing. The vegetables she used were like nothing I had ever seen before, with names I couldn't pronounce, let alone remember. She used seaweed—Jesus! The word itself made me queasy. Grains like millet and buckwheat were bandied about like we were all chirpy participants at an ornithological convention. Brownies and milk shakes began to flash through my mind like illicit pornography. My butt was getting numb, and I was becoming restless while the boring pudding made of watered-down apple juice and some crazy seaweed was handed out to all the students. Some of the participants were as annoyingly alive as the teacher, smacking their lips and cooing over the pathetic health-food Jell-O. I couldn't stand them.

One woman wore a turban to cover up what I assumed was chemotherapy-induced baldness. At the time, she gave me the creeps. I had heard that people came to macrobiotics to cure illness, but it just seemed too weird at the time. I know now, years later, that everything turns into its opposite: this woman, weak and pale, hanging on against all hope to the miso soup and the crummy pudding, was expecting to turn into our super–Homo sapiens teacher just by eating this weird food. And since then, I have seen that happen enough times to know that her faith was actually wisdom.

Class was finally over, and I got the hell out. So grateful to be spilled back into the throbbing, angry bloodstream of New York, I left the building alone, took a huge lungful of sour, metallic air, and relaxed.

But I had paid up front. For five classes. The ex-slacker in me was now into completing things, just for the sake of completing them, having left a small city of half-written papers, fruition-less world-saving strokes of genius, and dangling relationships in my wake. I may not have had cancer in my body, but I had a sort of behavioral cancer that even *I* knew about. It was a matter of pride to finish this out, just as an experiment in closure. Shoot.

I spent the next week enjoying cookies, ice cream, and the salty, oily specials at my local Polish diner. I jammed the photocopied recipe sheets I'd gotten from class into a crevice between the kitchen sink and the wall. When, after a short while, they got wet and blurry, I moved them to a hard-to-reach cupboard, demonstrating to myself my noble, newfound sense of responsibility.

Monday evening rolled around again, as it always seems to do, and suddenly my legs got very heavy. My butt was mysteriously soldered to the couch. Thick like peanut butter, thick like my sticky blood, resistance crossed its arms and stood before me like a frowning Mr. T. But I had to go. Hating every step, every second, every goddamned breath, I made my way back to the chrome-and-porcelain world of cooking class.

I sat down and did my best to avoid eye contact with the other students. The week's recipes were handed out. Hijiki! Daikon! Aduki beans?! Not again! If I wanted a trip to Japan, I thought, I'd buy a plane ticket! Ooooh, I was getting good and agitated, despising this and judging that. Miss Perfect Human Specimen glided in and sparkled up the room a bit. I wanted to kill her. I wondered whether the sentence for her murder would be harsher than normal, given her elevated humanocity. I didn't care. I'm sick of your millet with squash. Get lost with your split-pea soup! If you try to get another ridiculous excuse for a dessert past me tonight, you've got one coming!

Having never displayed any violent tendencies in my life (with the exception of one little spitting, scratching, lit-match-throwing catfight with my older sister while on vacation in Barbados), I wasn't sure what I was actually planning to do here. So I just let my inner T get off on saying "I pity the fool who tries to mock me with a wimpy, woody, health-food dessert! I pity the fool. . . ."

You know the ending to this story. You know that, somewhere along the line, I got hooked. Somewhere between the hiss of the pressure cooker and the nutty smell of the crushed sesame seeds, I was a goner. Mr. T took off his gold chains and just slipped away.

You see, the energy generated in that room by that natural food was clearer, crisper, and more electrified than what I was channeling in my own life. My apartment felt sludgy. My personality felt sludgy. I was only twenty-one, so my body felt only mildly sludgy, but I knew it was just a matter of time, observing all the sludged-up elders around me. And although my ego despised these clean, light vibes, because it knew they were going to shine a flashlight on all its baloney, my soul was utterly, utterly seduced.

Because this sparky, lightning vibe that is inside all of us is invisible, silent, and untouchable, it is impossible to describe. But it is definitely feel-able. As I ate macrobiotic foods, the sludge began to melt away, and the lightning sparks whipped through me. I had more energy than I had had since childhood. My skin felt soft, like a kid's. Pockets of fat, which had never before budged for a sit-up or a Diet Coke, began to melt away.

But more than that, the energy the food imparted was sustainable and even.

My moods began to stabilize. I wasn't freaking out at things that would have made me crazy before. I started to feel really connected to nature for the first time in my life because, as the spark fired through me, it resonated with other channels of this force, namely trees, flowers, and birds. New York City buses started to seem like humongous, dirty aliens, having no connection to anything organic.

People seemed to me the weirdest things of all: part spark, part sludge. I began to see people as organisms fighting to express, to release, to breathe energetically through all their sludge. And as mine melted away, theirs became doubly apparent to me. I was feeling like a little alfalfa sprout, so fresh and alive, while the people around me were overcooked pot roasts stuck in the pan.

And the cooking itself was getting interesting. I found that when I was in physical contact with these natural foods—especially grains—I calmed down. My mind cleared instantly, concentrating itself on the task at hand, like an effortless moving meditation. And another thing: I felt too afraid to tell anyone that I was sure—swear to God—that it was the grain, that little grain of rice (or barley or millet) that was reeling me in; it was doing all the work, not me. All I did was show up and let it work through me. But that just seemed too crazy.

I was learning how to cook the foods with spark. Not spark like a double espresso or a line of cocaine, but spark like the twinkly snow on a moonlit December night. Spark like the buzzy crickets of August. Spark like the thunderbolt of energy that shoots through you when a new lover draws near. The spark of life.

It is the energy that is flowing through you now, holding this book, reading these words. You can either push it down, inviting it to sneak out in weird and neurotic ways, or surrender to its laws and let it reveal the goddess that you are.

There is no right or wrong way to approach this book. One of the things I love about macrobiotics is that there is a food component and a philosophy component—theory and practice tucked side by side on your fork. You can start with your brain or with your belly.

This book is formatted in "phases" that sketch out a reasonable path for a person to follow, but may not be your destiny at all. You may want to jump straight to a desludging diet tomorrow or just read some of the philosophy over brown rice and see what happens next. Either way, you will learn what you are meant to learn on your personal timetable. I believe that if you are intrigued at all by either the cooking or the theory, then your intuition will guide you like a benevolent dominatrix.

part one

life lessons: the 12 laws of change of the infinite universe

After taking macrobiotic cooking classes for a while, I began to listen to the philosophy underlying the food; while casually chopping carrots, my teachers were talking about huge, ridiculous things like the universe and the galaxies. What a grain of rice had to do with my relationship to eternity, I had no idea. But I just kept chewing and listening, and slowly some little cosmic puzzle pieces clicked into place.

I began to understand that if you want inner freedom, peace of mind, and a healthy, beautiful body, it's important to understand the fundamental forces of the universe. These forces, yin and yang, are creating the natural world, your body, the food you eat, and everything else in your environment. By recognizing and understanding yin and yang, you can make food and lifestyles choices that help you harmonize with the bigger picture. And when you "tune in" to the greater whole, freedom and happiness will follow you like puppy dogs.

Since you are made of yin and yang forces, you have the ability to sense the yinness and yangness of things. After every law, I have included exercises for your "inner compass" to help you sense the world from the yin/yang energy plane. As you go "macro," eating whole and natural foods, your inner compass will become more and more accurate and dependable, and soon you will function freely from a healthy, clear intuition all the time. Yay!

CHAPTER ONE

laws 1, 2, and 3

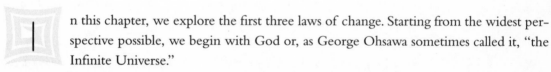 n this chapter, we explore the first three laws of change. Starting from the widest perspective possible, we begin with God or, as George Ohsawa sometimes called it, "the Infinite Universe."

This abundant source of all energy and things expresses itself through two forces, yin and yang, in its endless creation. Yin force is expansive and produces certain qualities in nature, foods, and people, while yang force is contractive and produces the opposite qualities in the world.

Yin and yang are IT—the whole enchilada. Every single thing in the universe can be seen through the lens of these opposites, expansion and contraction: nature, humans, ideas, art, relationships, sports, history, politics, religion. When this simple template is used for understanding the world, layers of confusion and concept fall away. But, most important, by understanding yin and yang, you can learn to cook in order to support your health physically, emotionally, and spiritually. Let's go!

law #1: one infinity manifests itself into complementary and antagonistic tendencies, yin and yang, in its endless change

Let's break this down into chunks. First, George Ohsawa called "One Infinity" the "infinite pure expansion." This is not the space we're floating in right now, but the spaceless origin of space. It is the oneness from which everything arises and to which everything returns. In his inimitable way, George Ohsawa liked to call it the "beginningless beginning and the endless end."

Shoot. We've already stumbled upon the ultimate ideological question: Do you believe in "One Infinity"? Do you have a name for it? Is it in the form of a person? A great spirit? Have you assigned it certain qualities? Or do you dismiss this concept out of hand? How do you relate to it? Do you believe in "energy" or scoff at your friend's feng shui crystals?

I didn't grapple with the idea of an infinite dimension infusing and underlying everything until the VISA card maxed out. I was fifty pounds overweight, and nothing was working the way my nice Torontonian parents had told me it would. Fame refused to land on my doorstep. Fortune seemed to fly away from me with the exact same speed that cookies mysteriously flew into my mouth. Sometimes, in the vast expanse of the night, I felt suicidal. If my navel was all there was to ponder, into eternity, no wonder we had invented TV. I started considering that maybe, just maybe, there was a world beyond the visible—a weird, bewitching dimension that held a meaning beyond my compulsive trek from deli to nightclub to aerobics class. Perhaps—God forbid—the parents were wrong.

As far as I am concerned, it doesn't matter the form or shape that this entity takes, as long as you acknowledge a source bigger than yourself. Although we have been told that it is so huge and mighty that it is impossible to truly comprehend, George Ohsawa believed that it was actually alarmingly simple. The purpose of this book is to help you sense and relate to the Infinite Universe by learning its laws and bringing your body back to its natural balance. Through macrobiotic practice you will regain your common sense.

non credo

But wait: George Ohsawa told his students never to believe a thing he said. He was very fond of a concept called Non Credo, meaning "I do not believe" in Latin. He thought that to be a living, breathing organism, hooked up to the Infinite Universe like everyone else, our experiences and intuition would give us all the lessons we need from our greatest teacher—the Infinite Universe. To believe blindly, without "discovering," was to be a slave, so one must go out (and in) to find the truth, never borrowing it cowardly from another. You didn't take your girlfriends' sordid stories about steamy Buicks and pimply adolescent shoulder blades as a substitute for your own experience of sex, did you? Of course not. You dove right in and found out for yourself. Well, one could argue that this God stuff is at least as important as that. So if you do not believe that there is one unity creating, animating, and uncreating the material world, test it for yourself. Argue with me. Argue with this book. Look around and find the evidence or lack thereof. Ask yourself how your hair grows and intestines glurg away, without your effort, thought, or direction. Where is all that energy coming from? What is its source? What pushes the moon to control the tides to lap at your toes on the beach? After eating whole grains for a while (which are themselves natural and united), your perceptions may change. Have fun. Live. Don't be a slave to this book, or any other. In macrobiotics, to learn and explore as a free being is encouraged. Discover for yourself.

Before we move on, here's a little tip: it helps to think of this source as neither benevolent nor malevolent, for it is beyond both. As the source of all things, it is both life-giving and life-withdrawing, and its laws are just, steadfast, and crystal clear. As you learn them, you will find that working with the Infinite Universe brings freedom and working against it brings suffering. By practicing macrobiotics you will polish your inner compass, which is your tool to align with the Infinite Universe, and the rest of your life is about buffing it to a shine and following its direction.

If the God of your childhood was vengeful, you might want to rename it the "Infinite Universe" for a while and keep an open mind about Its characteristics.

Hopefully, you will begin to see that this Infinite Universe—regardless of the temper of your "God"—makes room for lots of play. Nature, left to its own devices, is abundant, creative, and just.

So we're beginning with the assumption that there is this infinite source and that it presents as "One." You can call it God, Goddess, Allah, Brahman, P. Diddy, or Great Spirit. I tend to call it the Infinite Universe, but I'll also refer to it as God. The point is that we connect to something eternal and just, no matter the name it goes by. This book is about relating to this source in a healthy way.

Chunk two reads, "Manifests itself into complementary and antagonistic tendencies, yin and yang." Here we see that infinity—although it's actually "one"—presents itself to us as two. Tricky little universe. And these two are the nuts and bolts of creation.

Many religions seek to explore the relationship between what is considered the divine and the relative, material world of duality. There are various interpretations: from a great Oneness (Brahman, God, Allah) comes duality, whether that is interpreted as literal twosomes or simply the individual's separateness from God and others. The Bible opens up with "In the beginning, God [Infinite Universe] created the Heaven and the earth [yin and yang]," which is the Judeo-Christian introduction to duality. He then goes on to create many other dualities such as darkness and light, water and land, animal and vegetable, man and woman, blond and brunette. And the whole creative process is followed by its complementary opposite, a well-deserved rest.

This is the great paradox of our lives; we live in a world that we experience in a dual way; a world of opposites. And yet there is a great Oneness that creates and uncreates everything from behind the scenes and between our cells.

As creations of this oneness, we feel a natural pull to align with it. But our egos, from which we negotiate the material world, tend to be dualistic, limited, and self-centered. So we need assistance: spiritual pursuits are designed to help us remerge with this divine, creative life force. We meditate, partake in religious fellowship, or do service in order to bypass the ego and leap into the dimension of unity, where the soul hangs out and parties.

In macrobiotics, this fundamental paradox of spirit and ego—like all others—is happily embraced. By acknowledging this first law of the universe, we juggle the Oneness and duality of all things. However, instead of naming every single pair of opposites in the material world, we use Taoist terminology that identifies the essential tendencies underlying each pair; these tendencies are called yin and yang.

This dynamic duo is described as "complementary and antagonistic opposites." In English, the word *antagonistic* is normally construed as negative; it conjures bitchiness and catfights. The antagonist in a movie tends to be the guy holding a knife to Keanu's throat, and our lovely hero feels compelled to destroy the enemy. But within macrobiotic philosophy, all antagonisms are complementary, generating spark and energy. It is the way your competitor triggers a pissed-off, passionate urge to grow in your gut. Or an attractive member of the opposite sex being near you ignites sparks throughout your whole body. It is the pull between opposites, the charge found in difference. The Tao.

The third chunk is "in its endless change." Everything changes over time. We experience change within a day, a week, a year. We see great flux within our lifetimes, going from teen to grandma in what seems like the blink of an eye. Even plutonium, with a half-life of a bizillion years, does have a half-life. Civilizations rise and fall. Boyfriends come and go. And although they say that Twinkies will last a very, very, very long time, even their form is not eternal.

EXERCISE YOUR INNER COMPASS

Do you believe in an underlying creative force, or "God"?

If so, is this God faraway and detached from you, or do you feel a part of It?

How are men and women both antagonistic and complementary at the same time? How about liberals and conservatives? Sickness and health?

law #2: yin and yang are produced infinitely, continuously, and forever from the infinite pure expansion itself

In other words, "There's no gettin' outta this one." Although we might like to transcend duality completely, the Infinite Universe is chugging away, creating yin and yang tendencies endlessly in order to keep everything moving and changing.

Yet we seem to want to stop this ride and get off. Many religions have produced the idea of panaceas existing for us after this life, places where we can finally put on our jammies and kick back for eternity. But this law is claiming that the Infinite Universe is always moving, and as manifestations of it, so are we.

None of us is stopping. Getting older, wiser, or sexier, we are constantly being created and uncreated by the Infinite Universe itself, sloughing off cells with each facial and growing spiritually with every prayer.

Of course, the ego bristles against this concept, feeling its sovereignty threatened. This endless movement challenges every single thing's existence, pushing it to change, then change again, ad infinitum . . . literally.

But George Ohsawa, having surrendered to this reality, decided that the only reasonable approach to the situation was to "play." His theory was that if you've gotta sit around in the Duluth airport for all of eternity, you might as well have fun. He believed that a firm understanding of the laws of yin and yang, along with a healthy mind and body, could allow the individual to experience this eternal movement as a fabulous, fun adventure as opposed to a dreary life sentence. Some said life was suffering, but our boy "G" didn't buy that. Instead, he saw such flux within reality, and so much possibility within that flux, that suffering just seemed like one aspect of human experience. More precisely, by applying the laws of yin and yang, he saw all suffering become joy and all joy become suffering. Nothing was staying fixed for long, when perceived from eternity. By perceiving the complementary opposites in any phenomenon, you open the door to "play."

Many people who practice meditation, yoga, or other spiritual disciplines are looking to merge with the divine. But sometimes people become addicted to their spiritual practices in an attempt to permanently transcend the material plane they consider so chaotic. Macrobiotic practice approaches life this way: by eating whole grains and vegetables, and chewing them well, we are dropped effortlessly into the moment, feeling peace and calm. Macrobiotic foods help us to harmonize with the rhythms of the Infinite Universe, and from this vantage point we can recognize the complementary antagonistic opposites everywhere. When yin and yang are identified in every circumstance, and the laws of change are recognized, all material conflicts make sense. So-called "chaos" has identifiable causes and patterns. So instead of trying to transcend the whole scary mess of life, we can dive right in and play.

Regardless of what they eat, some people have already found ways to play happily in the river of continual manifestation: Nelson Mandela, Donald Trump, and Oprah Winfrey have all demonstrated their capacities to adapt to, and learn from, the ebb and flow of change within their lives.

And let us not forget America's first lady of change, Madonna. First we saw her shift from image to image with the flexibility of the wind, enjoying the flux and play of change faster than we could handle it. Each new wave of shock and criticism we lobbed at her seemed only to make her stronger, as struggle naturally should. Then it became clear that she was experiencing deep, personal transformation which she was unafraid to share with the world. This required great humility, faith, and self-esteem all at the same time. Instead of stagnating, which is our cultural synonym for aging, Madonna seems to be getting deeper and wiser, following the actual dictates of the Infinite Universe. A perpetual mold-breaker, she is like the Tibetan monk who spends months creating a complicated sand mandala with meticulous, concentrated devotion, and then sweeps it away in an afternoon.

It is understood in Buddhism that craving produces misery. In other words, getting too attached to the yin or yang of any situation sucks. Waiting desperately by the phone sucks. Believing that those five extra pounds are ruining your life sucks. George Ohsawa used a very specific word for this kind of attachment: *slavery*. We must remain flexible and playful, learning the laws of yin and yang because spending one's precious life attaching to the extremes of good and bad, us and them, or rich and poor becomes totally exhausting and ultimately fruitless.

However, allowing ourselves to perceive and identify with the unity *creating* our dualistic reality brings inner peace. But don't assume this means a lonely life with a shaved head and an ugly pair of sandals. On the contrary, from this perspective, we can indulge in the play of duality, enjoying the endless games of yin and yang without becoming enslaved by them. That is truly a big life. As big as Madonna's, or Gandhi's, or . . . Camilla Parker Bowles's. And what we eat can take us there.

EXERCISE YOUR INNER COMPASS

How do you feel about change?

What makes some changes "good" and other changes "bad"? What role does attachment play in your relationship to change?

Identify three big changes you have been through in the last five years. How did you adapt to them? Do you lean on friends or family, get spiritual, or eat chocolate chip cookies to handle the stress?

law #3: yin is centrifugal; yang is centripetal. yin produces expansion, lightness, cold, darkness. yang produces constriction, weight, heat, light

Now we're getting down to the nitty-gritty. As the earth spews outward, its lava blood busting through the cracks, expansive, yin force is dominant. Bubbles rising in a champagne flute, the sprouting of a seed, and a mad rush of blood to the cheeks are all examples of the upward, outward, centrifugal force that runs half our reality. It is holding us up right now. Without it, we would all be mushed hopelessly against the sidewalk, unable to take a step, let alone leap for joy.

Centripetal force is the exact opposite: a fist closing, a flower drooping, or your trash compactor squeezing a hunk of garbage. Any time contraction is occurring, yang force is predominant.

Wherever yin and yang come together, a spiral of energy is created. And spirals are everywhere; from the twisted corkscrew of the galaxy, to the dirty water spinning down your bathtub drain, the natural world expresses itself through spirals: the earth spins like a top around the sun. Tornadoes, ocean currents, and Stevie Nicks are all manifestations of spiraling energy. From the hair spiral on the top of your head, through the funky coils of your fingerprints, all the way down to your DNA, you are made up of spirals, too. And as a member of the spiral club, you are being created and uncreated by the Infinite Universe every moment of every day. Macrobiotics is about eating in order to align with this larger reality.

On every part of the planet, contracting yang force (also called heaven's force) is coming in from the cosmos, and yin, expanding force (also called earth's force) is exiting the earth. But depending on where you are situated on the planet, the ratio of yang cosmic vibes and yin earth vibes will vary. A person living near the North or South Pole is closer to the entry of the yang spiral coming in, so she receives much more contracting force than a person living in the Caribbean, who—being nearer the equator—is bathed in expansive earth vibes year-round. Those of us who live in the temperate zone have a mixed bag: during spring and summer, we experience more expansion, and in fall and winter we are governed by contraction. For everyone, eating in a way that harmonizes with the external environment is a key component to health and freedom. Although the macrobiotic diet is generally centered around the principal food of grain, it varies widely depending upon where the eater lives. In colder climates, more animal food, longer cooking times, and other yang factors may be necessary to harmonize with the environment. In warmer climates, lighter cooking styles, more tropical fruit, and other yin factors prevail.

As we look at these two more closely, we see that every single thing we deal with in our daily lives can be examined in terms of its yinness and yangness. Table 1 lists the different qualities that yin and yang produce in the world. I recommend you dog-ear this page and refer to it whenever you forget which is which.

THE YIN AND YANG OF HUMANS

Yin and yang not only enter the planet; they also enter our bodies. Ever hear your yoga teacher talk about chakras? Well, she's not crazy. As heaven's force rains down upon your head and the earth's force issues up from the earth, yin and yang collide to make seven spirals along the midline of your body. Each chakra (which means "wheel" in Sanskrit) radiates life force into your body and

TABLE 1: ATTRIBUTES CREATED BY EXPANSION AND CONTRACTION

ATTRIBUTE	YIN	YANG
Tendency	Expansion	Contraction
Function	Diffusion Dispersion Separation Decomposition	Fusion Assimilation Gathering Organization
Movement	More inactive, slower	More active, faster
Vibration	Shorter wave and higher frequency	Longer wave and lower frequency
Direction	Ascent and vertical	Descent and horizontal
Position	More outward and peripheral	Inward and central
Weight	Lighter	Heavier
Temperature	Colder	Hotter
Light	Darker	Brighter
Humidity	Wetter	Drier
Density	Thinner	Thicker
Size	More expansive and fragile	More contractive, harder
Form	Longer	Shorter
Texture	Softer	Harder
Atomic particle	Electron	Proton
Elements	N, O, P, Ca, etc.	H, C, Na, As, etc.
Climatic effects	Tropical climate	Colder climate
Biological quality	More vegetable quality	More animal quality
Sex	Female	Male
Organ structure	More hollow and expansive	More compacted and condensed

ATTRIBUTE (CONT.)	YIN (CONT.)	YANG (CONT.)
Nerves	More peripheral, orthosympathetic	More central, parasympathetic
Attitude, emotion	More gentle, negative, defensive	More active, positive, aggressive
Work	More psychological and mental	More physical and social
Consciousness	More universal	More specific
Mental function	Dealing more with the future	Dealing more with the past
Culture	More spiritually oriented	More materially oriented
Dimension	Space	Time*

*Adapted from *The Book of Macrobiotics,* by Michio Kushi (Japan Publications, 1987)

out to the world. Good health and happiness depend upon the yin-to-yang charge of your body's spirals being natural and balanced.

Each of your body's functions has its yin and yang phases; your heart, beating every second of your life, contracts and expands, delivering blood to your body and receiving it back when it is used. Your lungs are constantly expanding and contracting. As a woman, you contract and expand within your menstrual cycle. Your stomach, colon, and bladder all expand, thus accommodating food or its by-products, and when the time is right, they contract to expel them.

THE YIN AND YANG OF FOOD

Now let's look at vegetation. Imagine a garden, with rows of different vegetables. Put on your expansion-and-contraction glasses to see what's really going on here. First there is a leek, which grows up directly, its straight green leaves expanding to the left and right. All these qualities (up, green, expanded) are manifestations of expansive force coming from the earth. The yang force of the leek, most expressed in the root system, is weak relative to its upper body. Therefore, the leek is governed by yin. Upward-growing vegetables such as these energize the upward parts of the body—the liver, lungs, heart, and brain. In macrobiotic cooking, yin—upward-growing vegetables—are used to keep us feeling light and fresh.

The second row contains carrots. The feathery greens of a carrot are flexible and soft yet strong enough to allow us to yank on them to expose the orange root of the plant. When we bite it in half, we expose a distinct, tight spiral which is the root's core. All these qualities (hard, downward-growing, orange, tightly coiled) are examples of yang force. Therefore, the carrot is governed by yang. The "roots" of our bodies are our intestines and legs. Foods like carrots, parsnips, and burdock—especially when cooked for a long time—deliver heat, intestinal strength, and a feeling of rootedness to the planet.

In the third row we see cabbages. Round and heavy, they sit squat on the earth. In fact, peel back a few external leaves and their shape resembles the im-perfect sphere of the earth, which tells us that cabbages are made up of a ratio of yin to yang that mirrors that of the planet as a whole. Between the yin of the leek and the yang of the carrot, cabbage appears more "balanced." Round veg-etables such as onion, squash, and cabbage impart a sweet and soothing energy to the middle organs of the body, especially the stomach, spleen, and pancreas. In macrobiotic cooking, they are used to balance us, bringing us back to our center.

Eating foods that contain this natural order of contraction and expansion not only strengthens your health but also hooks you up with the larger whole; your cells literally resonate with the big picture. Your body finds its perfect weight, spiritual alignment feels effortless, and natural beauty—great hair, glowing skin, and inner radiance—results from this simple connectedness with nature. This is the fundamental difference between macrobiotics and any other "diet."

EXERCISE YOUR INNER COMPASS

The first part of this exercise is eating a cup of brown rice (see recipe, p. 83) and chewing every mouthful one hundred times. That may sound crazy, or even impossible, but do your best; the more you chew the rice, the more sensitive you will become to energy. To make the chewing easier, you can take a tiny bit of sauerkraut or pickle (unsweetened) with each mouthful. This will help to create lots of saliva and break down the rice. To learn more about chewing, go to p. 80.

After chewing, relax and take a few deep breaths. Now let your eyes have a fuzzy focus. In your mind, say the word *expansion,* and sense, around the room, all the ways in which objects are upward, outward, inflated, or long. Don't think. Don't judge. Just sense expansion, in any way that it comes to you. There may be only one thing in the room that screams "expansion" to you, or you may feel it everywhere. Both are fine. There is no right or wrong here; you are simply developing your inner energy compass.

Close your eyes and take a nice cleansing breath. When you open them again, let the focus be fuzzy and say to yourself *contraction,* and simply sense how things are tight, dense, small, and compact. Feel the closing energy in the room. Don't think. Don't judge. Just allow yourself to tune in to contraction. You may see contraction now in things that looked expanded before. That's great. Everything has both. Just exercise your inner sense.

Now go to the kitchen and get a vegetable. Place it on the counter. Relax and check out its yinness and yangness. Look at it solely in terms of expansion (how is it upward, outward, releasing?) and contraction (how is it downward, hard, or gathering?). If it is a root vegetable, examine carefully the place where the root and the tops meet. This is the point of most dynamic energy, and it is the lucky person who gets to eat it.

Try this exercise outside. Note the expansive qualities of a tree. The grass. A flower. Now sense the contracting force in them all. Notice how your body reacts to sunshine. Do you expand or contract? How about a cool breeze or snow?

Finally, after feeling the rice feeling for about an hour, warm up a cup of apple juice and begin to sip it. Drink at least half of it and see how you feel. Do you feel more expanded or contracted? How is this feeling different from before?

Phew! Let's take a freakin' break!

· Snack Break ·

I just went to Quebec City with a friend's kids, aged six and four, and I totally lost it. Upon entering Canada, usually right at the border, I have a tendency to regress to childhood. All it takes is a distance sign in kilometers, a paper-thin quarter with the head of Her Majesty and the tail of a moose, all wrapped up in an Anne Murray song to swing me right back into the seventies—when chocolate bars were dinner, or at least a daily aperitif. On the subway going home from school, there were days when I had three. The labels, with their golden, shiny promise of the sweet, sweet river of chemical bliss, had branded themselves on my subconscious mind. I had formed relationships with them, just as the manufacturers had hoped I would.

Now, as I passed racks of candy in the tourist shops we entered, the kids fighting over giant pencils covered in fleurs-de-lys, I played it cool, nonchalant, hard to get. A resident alien of the United States, green card in hand, I didn't need my sweet friends pathetically stuck in the tundra above the forty-ninth parallel. I fingered the little Châteaux Frontenacs encased in glass balls with falling snow. I had moved on to better things, like Hershey bars and Butterfingers. I had even moved beyond my new American candy-bar friends, to real food like soup and bread. Gone were the days of stuffing Crunchie bar after Coffee Crisp down my gullet, melted crumbs of sponge toffee glistening on my sticky down coat. I lived in a country now with actual *heat,* generated by the *sun,* allowing its people to come out of doors to eat cooling foods like salads and sprouts! I could relax now, the days of silent subway munching over and done. So there!

But I was fooling myself, *bien sûr.* Each time I passed the candies, the labels whispered to my subconscious mind like a skilled hypnotist: "You will eat me," they hissed, instantly compounding the thousands of experiences I had had doing just that. I could imagine what these chocolate bars looked like naked, their wrappers peeled back like hotel bedspreads in the evening. My mouth began to leak. I was nothing more than a hardwired network of responses ready to explode. I was a Canadian binge waiting to happen.

Plus, kids are intense. By day two of the trip, I bobbed like a broccoli stalk in the melty ice water of a picked-over vegetable tray while pretending to have fun with the kids in the pool. After about ten minutes, my limbs were numbing and my mind was wailing, "I haaaaate this!" My vegan-ish diet and deep inner life were no help to these children. They didn't need a Tibetan monk for a play-mate. Nor were they interested in my *big* perspective and spiritual solutions to all the messy things that grownups seem to get themselves into. Did these little shavers want to sit down for a civilized hour and tell me all about their prob-lems? No. These kids were busy tying all the knots that someone like me would eventually help them to pick at. What they needed now was a hot-blooded grownup, floating on a Styrofoam noodle, spitting chlorinated water right back at them.

I needed the sugar just to keep up.

Like a coked-up Mike Myers, I dove right in. First the Crunchie bar, a long and elegant log of sponge toffee covered in fine milk chocolate. If you suck on it patiently, the chocolate melts . . . slowly and willingly . . . eventually giving way to the harder, crunchier toffee, which, left to its own devices, would rip up the roof of the mouth like dry Cap'n Crunch. So the sponge toffee must be nuzzled, held, and wooed. And then, just when it all feels useless and you're ready to give up and bite down hard, the spongy, airy toffee simply implodes, like a mound of shaving cream disintegrating in your hand. It almost seems to disappear completely when your tongue discovers the alchemical miracle of this Canadian coup; the sponge toffee has morphed into a hard, chewable, stick-to-your-teeth candy that the tongue will chase for hours as it hides like a sneaky lit-tle devil between molars and gums. Yang becomes yin becomes yang.

Suddenly, I was good to go with the kids. I was singing silly songs, crawling on top of eighteenth-century cannons, and pointing out the funny *chapeaux* of passing French ladies. This was what they needed—a souped-up, overheated, nonstop talking fun machine! I had all the patience in the world, translating words like *street* to *rue,* helping them to remember it by imagining Pooh's mar-supial friend Roo hopping down the boulevard! God, I was good! My frontal lobe throbbed with blood and energy and ideas. Life was suddenly *upthisclose* to my face, instead of a broad horizon of Taoist balancing acts played out over eter-nity. Forty-five minutes was now "one episode of *Arthur*" and "half an episode of *Dragon Tales,*" which seemed quite pleasant and manageable. All I had to do was not think about myself, and the growing hole that the chemicals and sugar were burning inside of me. Just think about the kids. Be here for the kids. Aim the energy at the kids. And when it all comes crashing in on you, eat another chocolate bar.

So I did. A Caramilk bar, some Smarties, and a Coffee Crisp later, we were off to dinner. The truth be told, I had no interest in real food anymore, anything that had come out of the earth seeming sort of dead and tasteless. I just needed some salt. Something to contract my canker-ridden lips back to normal. Pull my brain back from the preschool precipice. Stop the room from spinning so I could settle back into what used to be my nervous system. I ordered pasta with smoked salmon. That sounded nice and salty, and a Caesar salad, lots of croutons, lots of anchovies, hold the lettuce.

The sugar was doing its thing. My face looked bloated, and my thighs had a distinctly premenstrual feel in the middle of the month. The blood vessels in my eyes were redder than usual, the surface of the balls glassy. I was a heat machine, extra calories pumping their way out every pore. Although normally I felt cool at night, the single fleece blanket on the bed seemed too much, and I had to poke both feet, one knee, and most of my upper body out from under it. Un-concerned about any of these little inconveniences, my life having become a joyous living sacrifice to *the kids,* I will concede that I was grateful to lie down at last that night. What a surprise to discover that, although my muscles were happy to stop, my brain was not. "Why aren't you married?" "What are you do-ing with your life?" "You're a loser." "You are ugly." Instead of counting sheep, I racked up self-defeating thoughts. I tried meditating on my breath, under-standing full well that it was the sugar making me miserable, but as soon as I reeled in my mind for one inhalation, it went dancing out the door again, play-ing with the Halloween hobgoblins of my soul. "You left your country." "You don't belong anywhere." "You'll never finish your book." "It sucks anyway."

I tossed and turned, in a failed attempt to shake these S&M thoughts from my brain. Or were they M&M thoughts? It was no use. The sugar was making its way out, like a vampire leaving the coffin to party in the dark. It was an ex-treme energy, chattering, spinning, exploding as it exited my mellow grain-and-vegetable body, and my only choice was to just sit through it. I had done it before and I could do it once more. I embarked on my sweet dreams with a cheerful round of "I'll never eat sugar again!"

Right. The next morning, hungover and craving a hair-of-the-dog-that-bit-me, I stumbled down to the hotel brunch buffet, complete with buttery, pre-mapled crepes and rainbow-colored cereal. I just gave up. I knew the trip would last only one more day and then I would back in my life, cooking pots of rice and thinking carrots were actually sweet.

So I indulged again, throwing every sound nutritional principle I knew into the St. Lawrence River, watching them float silently out to sea. This was my vacation, for God's sake. I deserved to have a little fun, a little misery, break some rules, *n'est-ce pas?* I drank a Labatt's and tried poutine, Quebec's contribution to the culinary world, consisting of french fries, gravy, and cheese curds. *Mmmmmm.* Before you could say *Bon appétit* my consciousness had exploded out of its lacquered, Asian box and made a big Western mess all over the weekend. I felt gloriously in tune with every North American, just barely making it from the Pepsi to the Dorito to the ice-cream cone. Barreling through a bunch of todays disconnected from any past or any future. Needing, needing, *needing* that "Quebec is for Lovers" T-shirt right this SECOND! Strolling down the promenade, gut leading with pride, owning the joint. I loved it. Forget spiritual growth. This is freedom.

And now I'm home. The roller-coaster ride is almost over. My friends are enduring the Chatty Cathy I have become as the last of the sweet stuff leaves my bloodstream. This story is a discharge, too. In a day or two, as the darkness creeps around, squeezing out every drop of seratonin from my brain, just before a new rush of it floods in, I will feel down, as if life is just not worth it. But I will not pick up a chocolate bar this time. I am in the States now. None of your sugary dreck calls to me. Thank God. I will sit through the darkness, knowing it will pass, as all things do, and come crawling back to the broad horizon, like a good little Taoist.

CHAPTER TWO

laws 4 and 5

n this chapter, we look at the mysteries of attraction and repulsion. From molecules to marriage, attraction plays its role to bring yin and yang together on every level of existence. Likewise, the repulsion that takes place when yang meets yang and yin meets yin determines (just as importantly) what we repel or reject in our lives. By understanding attraction and repulsion, you will begin to see these phenomena occurring everywhere you look. By sensing attraction and repulsion, you will become a masterful, magical cook. Hey, that rhymed!

law #4: yin attracts yang. yang attracts yin

Like lovesick teenagers from opposite sides of town, yin and yang always find a way to connect. But yin and yang don't simply attract each other; they literally depend upon each other for anything to exist within the Infinite Universe.

For example, yin electrons are attracted to yang protons to make atoms. Yin oxygen loves to interact with yang hydrogen, making water. Yang boys chase yin girls, making romance. The yang ovum attracts the yin semen, making people. The yang iron of our blood attracts the yin oxygen of the air, and, conversely, the yin chlorophyll of a plant's "blood" attracts the yang carbon dioxide of the air. We don't need to *decide* what to breathe; the law of attraction takes care of that!

We are being run by these forces. For example, you are sitting at a bar. There are salty chips in front of you. Bored, and waiting for your date, you take a few handfuls to pass the time. Very soon, you must have something to drink, whether it's just water or an alcoholic beverage. What just happened in terms of yin and yang? The salt causes contraction in the blood. This contracted blood (yang) attracts fluid (yin) from your mucous membranes and triggers a thirst signal in your brain. Feeling this dehydration, you order a drink to restore your fluids. You have no choice; in fact, you don't feel "right" until you've chugged some water.

Likewise, if you fill up on sweets at your kid's birthday party, all you want when you get home is some chicken salad, or salty pretzels, something to pull you back to center. These choices tend to go unnoticed, because they are happening on a purely mechanical level. As you behave intuitively, you are being used as an instrument of the Infinite Universe to restore balance.

We're all doing some form of this dance every day with food. That's why I like to say to people "You're already basically macrobiotic—you just don't know it!" It's just a matter of the extremes to which one is going. For instance, when animal food is ingested (strong yang), fruit, sugar, potatoes, tomatoes, or alcohol (all strong yin) is sure to accompany it. But this balance may be too stressful for the human body every day. Extreme yin attracts extreme yang, and we don't always want to bounce between extremes.

Alcoholics and drug addicts wonder why their lives become so hard; the answer is simple. The chronic ingestion of yin drugs (or alcohol) makes the condition of the nervous system extremely expanded and weak. This extreme yin naturally attracts extreme yang. A car crash is quick and hard (yang). Poverty is limiting and contracting (yang). Jail is the ultimate contraction of your life (yang). As long as the body is unnaturally expanded, the universe will offer up yang to make balance. When the yin drugs are thrown out, the body comes back to its center and life becomes less extreme.

Control freaks (yang) attract wimps (yin), and wimps attract control freaks. They may end up hating each other, but they stay together. Relationships like this end or transform only when one partner does some serious changing, thereby altering the cause (self), which changes the effect (marriage).

The attraction between Republicans and Democrats is what keeps American government moving. Knowing what you know already, which party do you think is more yin and which is more yang?

I cooked dinner one night for a friend in New York. After eating, I hesitated to tell her how I felt, because it just seemed too way-out. So I was stunned when she read my mind and said: "I don't know what you put in that meal, Jess, but I feel high." It was nothing more than yin and yang forces in their natural, food form. The electricity between them is real.

When yin meets yang, it often leads to a feeling of wholeness or harmony; a pleasing balance is struck. This is the satisfaction of eating a balanced meal, or creating a work of art, or making love. So we are intuitively making balance all the time; artists bring together dynamic opposites; chefs delight our palates with pleasing polarities; we try to fix up our single friends with people with whom they will "click."

In macrobiotic cooking, we are always seeking the dynamic charge between yin and yang. In a meal, we use upward-growing vegetables to balance downward-growing ones; wet comes with dry, crunchy with soft, and sea vegetables balance land vegetables. Warm colors balance cool ones, raw complements cooked, and hot strikes a dynamic friendship with cold. Where there is animal food, there is usually a dessert. The five tastes—pungent, sour, sweet, salty, and bitter—cover the journey between yin and yang. The more complementary antagonistic opposites you can include in a meal (or a day), the more dynamic it is for your health—physically, mentally, and spiritually.

EXERCISE YOUR INNER COMPASS

Where and when have you experienced strong attraction in your life? Attraction that is not conceptual (like "I should go there, I should do this") but attraction that feels like magnetism. What makes you walk across the room? What would make you fly across the country? Close your eyes and imagine a person you're REALLY attracted to. What happens in your body as he or she appears in your imagination? Is energy shifting? Is it subtle or pronounced? What does attraction feel like?

Imagine a natural food that you like or are strongly attracted to. Just relax and imagine this food. How does your body relate to the idea of that food? What is your inner compass doing? Now imagine your favorite "junk" food. Feel your attraction to it. Is it similar or different? Stronger or weaker? Does it make your mouth water? Eat a big dill pickle. What do you want next? What do you automatically start looking for?

Here's a slightly more complicated exercise: observe a couple in your circle of friends. In terms of personality, which partner is more yin and which is more yang? Who's more active and who's more laid-back? Understand that no person is all one energy, so there will be different yins and yangs within every relationship, but ask yourself: what are the qualities in each person that are attracted to the opposite in the other?

Practice identifying the attraction between yin and yang every day. As your intuition strengthens, you will be able to enter the kitchen "sensing" yin and yang, as opposed to thinking about them. It is this intuition that will direct your cooking, your health, and your happiness. Enjoy.

law #5: yin repels yin. yang repels yang

Meanwhile, there's a whole second story going on. We tend to be obsessed with attraction in our culture—we love wanting, needing, and getting. But what we often overlook is the rejecting, pushing, and losing that are happening all around us at the same time. There is as much repulsion as there is attraction in the universe, and it is totally natural. If there were no repulsion, everything would just be stuck in one huge galactic ball of rubber bands (actually, there would be nothing, but that's not as fun). By acknowledging and accepting repulsion, we experience more freedom.

I remember playing with magnets as a kid. The attraction between opposite poles was fierce; magnets snapping together as decisively as a Republican flicking the switch in a voting booth. But when I turned one magnet around, bringing the same poles close to each other, a funky repelling took place. This was one of my first lessons in the invisible world of energy. When I tried to jam the magnets together, ignoring the power of the repulsion, I could do it eventually, but it required much effort and was a willful violation of the way nature wanted the energy to flow. When I let go of my effort, the energy returned to its natural order.

Just as we exhale, we should let natural repulsion do its thing; when it's time to let go of something, let go. Don't hurl it across the room; just let it go. But because of our sludge, we tend to cling to things that are meant to slip away. Or worse, we tighten our grip crazily on something that is fighting to get away from us. Repulsion happens whether we like it or not. When we let repulsion play its role in life, it eventually runs its course, and we give it the chance to turn into attraction again.

Repulsion doesn't need to be dramatic; sometimes it's simply a lack of attraction. It's what's keeping us from marrying every single person we know and the force that keeps oil hovering over water.

Extreme yang versus yang repulsion usually results in some sort of explosion, like hooligans at a soccer game or two countries battling in war. Yin versus yin repulsion can be more subtle, like two depressed people who never meet because they're both locked away in their rooms. In chemistry, we see yin elements that bind with other yin elements only with the help of a yang catalyst. Likewise, yang elements get together with the help of a strong yin buddy.

Alcohol is always an illustrative example because it is an extreme: you've had a long, hard day and you're feeling tense and contracted (yang). You crave a cocktail (yin), which makes perfect energy sense because yang attracts yin. The first few sips feel wonderful, expanding your arteries, releasing your brain, relaxing your whole body. You sigh with appreciation. The rest of the cocktail tastes great, and so does most of the next. Depending on your original condition, it may take several drinks, but eventually you feel balanced; all the tension has disappeared, and now you are teetering on the yin side of the seesaw. You're becoming extremely yin and a little sloppy. You may be letting things slip that you would never admit sober. Your coordination is impaired, and you're getting tired. Hopefully you go home at this point. But if you don't and continue to drink, your body, which is now very yin, will repel any alcohol that it considers excessive by projectile vomiting it all over your buddies. This is nature's loving way of trying to teach you this principle: yin repels yin.

When I first practiced macrobiotics, I got extremely yang. I learned cooking only from books, most of which were written at a time when macrobiotics had a much saltier, Japanese bent. Having been addicted to sugar in the past, I was also firmly convinced that fruit, natural sweets, and other strong forms of yin were "bad." Instead of adapting the diet to my own life and environment, I continued to eat "by the book" and really overdid it on the salt, shoyu, and miso. I kept yangizing and yangizing myself without really knowing what I was doing.

I lost a lot of weight, so much so that people worried I had anorexia, although I was eating like a horse. I cut my hair short like a boy's; my condition was so yang that it squeezed out all the yin fat and hormones that would support menstruation, and I lost my period for a long time. My boobs deflated. I felt drawn to spiritual pursuits and quite above the material fray. Eating like a Japanese monk, I climbed up my own lonely mountain and sat in my own personal monastery in the middle of Manhattan.

Needless to say, my love life sucked. Monks aren't big daters. I felt little or no attraction to guys and they must have felt repelled by me, since I was basically turning into a boy. This was one of my strongest lessons in repulsion; yang repels yang. I kept complaining to my therapist that all my friends were either straight women or gay men, much to my confusion. I thought I wanted to be in a relationship, but it just wasn't happening.

This went on for quite a while, until I began to learn cooking from actual human beings who could communicate yin and yang to me in a way that related to my circumstances. Many of them were lovely, glowing, feminine women with curves in all the places I used to have them. They completely recognized the trap I had fallen into (many of them having done the same thing), and one even referred to me affectionately as the "pickle" because of all the salt I'd ingested. Among other things, they showed me that a dessert every day or so wouldn't kill me and that I could cut way down on the salt, the soy sauce, and the miso. I learned to "yinnize" my diet and let the natural expansion that governs a woman creep back into my body. I relaxed, filled out, and let the magnet flow the way it's meant to. Eventually, yin took over, and I attracted a lovely yang boyfriend.

Just as I could force the magnet to touch its similar pole, we make choices every day that violate the actual force field animating us. We eat "by the book." We marry people we're not deeply attracted to because they're "good people"; we hang out with people who actually repel us, feeling a responsibility to be polite. We go to jobs that crush us, day after day, because it's the "right thing to do." We deny ourselves our attractions—calling them sinful temptations—because we are afraid we will be enslaved by them.

We spend a lot of energy forcing similar magnetic poles to stay together. The tragedy is that not only are we wasting our own life force by trying so hard, what we are accomplishing is unnatural and in violation of the order of the universe. When we let go and surrender to the actual order, our egos may be miffed, but everyone ends up free in the end.

The more sludge we pack into our body, the less in touch we are with the actual magnetic force field we are a part of. The more natural food we eat (high in minerals and charged magnetically), the more we recognize natural attraction and repulsion and follow their lead. After eating macrobiotically for a while, you will sense your inner compass more and start to respond to these deep "pushes" and "pulls" from within your body.

In macrobiotic cooking, we make as many choices out of repulsion as we do attraction. For example, you cease to add salty seasoning to a dish when your intuition says, "Stop." This is yang repelling yang. Likewise, you stop adding liquid to a soup when your intuition shouts, "Enough." This is yin repelling yin. Without these moments of repulsion, cooking becomes out of balance.

EXERCISE YOUR INNER COMPASS

Close your eyes and imagine something that you hate, avoid, or reject. As you contemplate that thing or person, how is your body responding? Is it contracting or expanding? How is it different from attraction? Imagine a food that you have never liked. What happens in your body/mind as you imagine it?

It is natural for us to repel things. But what is the energy you recognize behind repulsion? Is it contraction or expansion? Or is it different depending upon the thing you are repelled by?

· McHeartbreak ·

I have just been dumped. Unceremoniously, unkindly, unwittingly dumped by six-foot-four, smooth-bodied Michael. Actually, when the facts are pored over in the future in the court of love, it will be clear that I did the official dumping, but only after having been treated so badly that no girl worth her gym membership would have any choice but to dump. He relied on a favorite of the North American male—the passive-aggressive breakup. I can just see it now, on the cover of *Esquire* and *Details* in bold and happy lettering: "Make her angry enough to dump YOU! Works like a charm!"

Unfortunately for me, I am a grain and vegetable eater. This means that I have feelings. But worse than that, I have unified thoughts. My mind will only go to "jerk" for about thirty seconds before it bounces back to "he's a frightened human being." You may think that this is simply the codependent denial of the typical female dumpee, but I assure you, it is more than that. I am always perceiving a front and a back, an inside and an outside, things morphing into their opposites within the bigger flux of change. Even this pain of the dumping, the grief that life is urging me to have seems simply the appropriate balance to the highs I got at the beginning. I am even compelled to acknowledge my responsibility for at least half of this anguish, having jumped in the sack with a good-looking guy way too fast—before I'd worked the "Rules" on him quite completely, establishing that he was hopelessly and pathetically in love with me, ring tucked in jockstrap, waiting to pop the question.

I made the mistake, as well, of projecting brown rice all over a Domino's pizza eater, seeing in his eyes as we made love the depths of the deepest oceans mixed with the strength of the mightiest mountain, when in fact, I was picking up the glaze of that morning's doughnut. Over time, none of this would have played out very well, and I see that now. My solid, steady grain-chewing self would have bored his frantic, bike-riding lothario, and the flame would have extinguished itself. Our differences attracted each other with incredible intensity, but that kind of attraction can become its opposite of repulsion in a heartbeat. Oh well. It was nice while it lasted. The warmth was real.

I am tired of these feelings. Tired of the grief and the loneliness that follow it like an annoying little orphan in a dirty dress. I am sick of balance and perspective, healing and growth. I don't want to surrender to this situation, feeling gutted like a fish on the sidewalk. At the same time, I don't want to "move on," "get over it," and "forget him." I can't. I am in this thing like a tender, silky flower, doing her best to press open the petals that were crushed by the big, careless ogre of a boy. My whole-foods existence keeps me locked in the perpetual now, patiently allowing my subconscious mind to sort through all the evidence and the sensations, the phone calls, and the kisses. Beneath my neck, it is recording and releasing, editing and augmenting. I am *processing* this situation, like a good Oprah fan, and I can't stand it.

This is a job for McDonald's.

I enter. The first thing I love about McDonald's is that, as in one's own home, it is not necessary to make a purchase in order to use the facilities. I have yet to have a polyester-clad McDonald's employee chase me down as I sneak into the bathroom off the highway. I love that. Too often, when I lived in Manhattan, I was struck with the panic of a full bladder in the face of thousands of bitchy New York restaurant owners wagging their fingers and spitting "Customers Only!"

But not at Mickey D's. Nooo way. This is America's home. It's as if, as I push open the door and am greeted by a greasy cloud of chemicals, I hear the whisperings of: "You grew up here. You've eaten Big Macs and supersized fries from here to Montana and back again. You've lived through McNuggets, McRibs, and McFlurries. You've kept your eyes on the fries for all these years and we love you. You're one of us. Go take a pee." So I do.

Refreshed and ready to order, I approach the counter. I can't get over how comforting it is to be in a McDonald's. The little hats. The funky cash registers that always looked so Space Age when I was a kid. The menu on the board above the heads of the workers. It's never a little booklet. Nor a card. Always the board. In fact, no one ever looks directly in the eye of a McDonald's employee while ordering. We squint above their heads, and they look at our Adam's apples all day. One is always looking up, rereading the selection exactly as it appears on the board. Just to make sure it's still there. Please, God, let it be there.

"A medium Filet-O-Fish meal with a Diet Coke, please." Eyes come down. Slightly embarrassed smile to balance the vulnerability of neck exposure. But she doesn't care. She is not here to shame me. She is here to serve me.

Ducats exchanged. Paper liner placed on tray. Followed by the blessed flurry of activity required to serve my needs. This is better than an expensive spa in the Berkshires! Michael may not want to show up for me, but, dammit, McDonald's does.

I choose the Filet-O-Fish because it sounds like Olde English. Gives the place a bit o' history, even if it's fake. Makes me want to put on an accent and become a whole new person in front of all my brothers and sisters here today. They wouldn't care. To them, I am everywoman, a nobody and a somebody all at once. I am brown and blue and gray, trekking in slush with the best of them, fading into the molded plastic seats until our allotted time is up.

But more than that, I don't think I could stomach a burger at this point. I may be a macrobiotic poseur, eating grains and veg regularly enough so I can "play" around with impunity, but those things simply aren't food. They are wet, leathery animal bits, fastened together with Ray-Kroc-only-knows-what and cooked just enough to achieve the color of office furniture.

But that's just my opinion now; I wouldn't have said any of that my senior year in high school when I bought a Big Mac every single day after typing class. Nor would I have poo-pooed the hotcakes and golden syrup during the spring that my best friend and I met daily for breakfast before school. And if lunch period were long enough that day, we could run over for some fries. God forbid I should have complained when my dad took my sister and me to McDonald's on the weekend mornings we spent with him. On those days, the Hamburgler games on the paper liner of the tray provided a perfect distraction from the nervousness I felt around my own flesh and blood. And perhaps I shall go back to my beloved burger, as a blue-haired old lady ordering from my Buick in the drive-thru. And when the coffee spills, scorching my girdle and marbled thighs, I shall not sue; no, I shall not sue. Besides, with the warnings on the cups nowadays, I wouldn't make a dime.

My tray is being assembled. Filet-O-Fish wrapped in its signature blue paper. We are now awaiting the fries. Of course, we all know that really means awaiting the loud and persistent beeping of the fry fryer over to the left, next to the fry bin where they are salted under the orange heat lamp and shoved through the metal scooper, which is open at one end and perfectly fitted to the red french fry box on the other. Who is not familiar with the professional and serious scooping action of the experienced employee, shoving arm down and then back toward the edge of the bin to get you the biggest, most neatly packed batch of french fries possible in that moment? And then the gentle and loving shaking down of the fries into the receiving box. It is a delicate maneuver that requires attention and care—more care than a certain Michael bothered to muster! They love me. I knew it.

And then the cup. A shock, really, considering I am expecting the McDonald's of Olde. It is empty. Completely empty. Which makes up only half of my surprise because it is also gigantic. I could shove my purse into it neatly. I asked for a medium Diet Coke and am presented with an enormous vessel of air. Since no one but me seems the least bit flummoxed by this strange reality, I become a little embarrassed by my ignorance. I want to ask, "What the hell is going on?" but instead, just pull my tray toward me along the counter and decide to wrestle privately, for a moment, with this puzzle. It hurts to think that everything changes. Even McDonald's. As I turn, I see the drink station on my right. Ahhh. Aha. I get it. I am being trusted to pour my own beverage! For a split second, it feels like Christmas Day in my bloodstream: I COULD GET A MILLION RE-FILLS pulses through me, igniting that inner thief I like to think we all have. Like a slimy guy on a winning streak at a huge Vegas casino, I dare to think: I AM GOING TO BEAT THE HOUSE. Never mind that an extra thirty-two ounces of chemicalized water will corrode my colon long before it'll topple the arches, the illusion feels great.

I choose a little eating nook near the windows. Having always been way ahead of the crowd on design, McDonald's boldly ushered in the weirdly shaped tabletops sometime in the '70s. Always smooth cornered so that no young foreheads get punctured in the fray, my table is affixed to the side of the restaurant, giving me a snug feeling of belonging between it and the plastic seat, also mysteriously born of the wall. I slide myself in and prepare to eat.

I can't believe they call that a bun. It is more like the soft, white mush of your great-aunt's cheek. Pasty, it dissolves in the mouth, becoming sticky and sweet. But this, of course, is the ingenious complement to the hot and greasy fish patty melting against the salty, sweaty cheese. And the tartar sauce, both creamy and tangy, completes the centerpiece of the meal. And it is a complete meal. The diet soda adds that slight bitterness of cola and the pungency of carbonation as it tickles your nose like wasabi. Sweet, sour, salty, bitter, and pungent. Cold and hot. Liquid and solid. Soft and hard (the well-cooked ends of the fries). This is the perfect feng shui of the Filet-O-Fish meal. We cannot escape the order of the universe. Even here.

Of course, I haven't come here for the taste; I have come here for the energy. I was looking for something to quiet the nerves, press "pause" on my inner movies, dull the brain. And it works. If I were allowed to use only one word in describing the food at McDonald's, it would be this: THICK. Everything is thick. Whether it's with oil or cheese or the mysterious ingredients of a "shake," it all ends up thick. And that is why I'm here. I want my blood thickened enough to slow down my circulation, to successfully impede the flow of energy to the overactive parts of my frontal lobe. Where there is wonder and curiosity and regret, I want sludge. Instead of weighing and measuring every thought with my delicate Taoist scales, I want a big, heavy sledgehammer pounding down like a judge's gavel proclaiming: he's an ass. Doing my best to avoid an afternoon of internal reflection and lip-biting tears, I want to settle into my larger role as a North American, fueled by this thick and warming chemical bomb that will propel me quite naturally into the mall where I will trudge through the aisles, fingering singing teddy bears and nail polish, putting it all on my trusty credit card with the satisfied resignation that "this is what we do."

Mission accomplished. I push away from my table, neither happy nor sad, just thick. I seem to have more physical energy than before, but my mind has slowed. The gray and sleety weather looks almost inviting to me now. Nothing's that bad. Get over it. He's a jerk.

I step out into the cold and hear the smack of my boots on the pavement. I am moving on, as part of the great collective, herding ourselves through the stores with cell phones like cowbells. We are a big family. We all eat at McDonald's, and we all go into debt at Christmas. The Michaels are the shiny, glass ornaments that get smashed on the floor when the tree comes down. Get over it. This is what we do. This is what we do. "Moooooooo."

CHAPTER THREE

laws 6, 7, 8, and 9

S o far, everything has been pretty simple: yin attracts yang; yang attracts yin—on some level; you already knew that. But now the laws of change get a little deeper and more specific. By studying very mechanical truths like "All Physical Manifestations are Yang at the Center and Yin at the Periphery," to laws that explain the incredibly complicated dynamics that occur within relationships and larger organisms, we are beginning to develop our macrobiotic minds. Don't feel that you need to understand this stuff like you are studying for a math test or a spelling bee; yin and yang will provide mental acrobatics for eternity, and the only test you have is your own life. Just read this information and see if it resonates within you. Eat whole grains for a year and read it again. Notice how it changes as you change.

law #6: nothing is solely yin or yang: everything is composed of both tendencies in varying degrees

This is an extremely important concept. Because our conscious minds are trained to look for antagonism within opposites, we are always looking for the good versus the bad, the right versus the wrong. Therefore, to perceive both yin and yang tendencies in all things can take some major mental readjustment.

It is very common for newcomers to macrobiotics to approach food with black-and-white thinking: "Carrots are yang. Leeks are yin." But each vegetable has yin and yang qualities. The carrot may be downward, hard, and orange (yang qualities), but it also is sweet and has upward-growing greens (yin). Meanwhile, the leek is green, upward, and expanded in its growth (yin tendencies) but is pungent when raw, relatively hard, and has downward-growing roots (yang). The carrot has more yang qualities than yin, and vice versa with the leek, but we certainly can't call a carrot "yang" and a leek "yin." This may seem petty in the beginning, but the habit of rigid classification can lead to real problems later on when you need to adjust your own condition.

Looking to our bodies, we have some yinner things and some yanger things. Thinking about expansion and contraction, the skin is very stretchy and expanded while the bones are very hard and contracted. Red blood cells are more contracted, white blood cells expanded. Some organs are solid and compact, others hollow and expanded. Wherever you see yin, look for yang. Wherever you see yang, look for yin. You will always find them both.

Sometimes it's hard to see. For instance, a rock seems pretty heavy and dense. Where is the yin there? Well, if the rock has any substance at all, there is some expansion keeping the elements from imploding into themselves completely. It may be that the rock is relatively porous. Some yin quality must be there in order for the rock to take up space in the material world. Air seems extremely yin, but even *it* has dynamic qualities. It is denser at sea level because its yang components fall toward the earth and thinner in the mountains where its yin components rise.

The more you eat whole foods, the more holistic your thinking will become. After a while the yins and yangs of things start leaping out at you, and you cease to believe that anything is simply one way.

If anything were to be solely yang, it would contract into nothingness. Likewise, pure expansion, untethered by yang energy, evaporates into nothingness. The earth could not exist if the yang spiral entering at the poles did not reverse itself into a yin spiral. Likewise, we would have no place to sit upon if it were made of only expansive force. So anything that we recognize as a phenomenon in the material world must be composed of both energies. And if you're a human being, that means you have both energies on physical, emotional, and mental levels, too. For example: your boyfriend may be tough on the outside—hard, strong, buff—with a serious look on his face, but a softie on the inside. Likewise, your best friend, always trying to drop the soft, expanded forty pounds she carries on the outside, can be steely hard on the inside.

EXERCISE YOUR INNER COMPASS

Cut an apple in half: now let's check out its yinness and yangness; where is it moist, and where is it dry? Which parts are expanded, and which parts are small and contracted? Where is it round, and where is it straight? Begin to identify expressions of contraction and expansion, noticing that they always come together. Now look at a human-made object, like your bed or a chair. What are its yang qualities (is it small, hard, warm, short, dense, angular, horizontal?), and what are its yin qualities (where is it large, expanded, soft, round, cool, tall?). There's no right or wrong here—you will always see both qualities. The goal is to begin to identify yinness and yangness in all things.

And don't forget, you're part of the material world, too: in what ways are you more yang (short, stocky, concentrated, active, social, controlling?) and in which ways are you more yin (tall, willowy, soft, receptive, depressive, artistic, dreamy?). Just as your parents' genes created a wacky mishmash inside of you, how are yin and yang showing up in you? What is your unique combination of qualities? Remember to look for both.

law #7: all physical manifestations are yang at the center and yin at the periphery

This law holds true because centripetal force creates the centers of things and centrifugal force creates the peripheries. All physical objects have a center, an energetic tether holding them together. In the human, our surface is made of skin, which is flexible, soft, and extremely expandable, clearly governed by yin. At our physical center is a skeleton, which is hard and contracted, clearly yang. As you begin your detective work, looking at the world in terms of yin and yang, this law will guide you in seeing how these two energies are always found working together, expanding and contracting to different degrees, holding up our material world.

One of the first clues to a macrobiotic counselor about the cause of a physical condition is its location in or on the body. Symptoms showing up on the upper body need different treatment than those showing up down below. Likewise, skin conditions are telling a different story than troubles lodged deep inside. Macrobiotic counselors consider how energy is moving in the body—where it is balanced, where it is excessive, where it is blocked—and treat the problems using yin and yang as their healing compass. It is fascinating to be seen by a macrobiotic counselor who peers at your feet, your eyes, and your hands, rather than staring at an X ray. Try it sometime.

With respect to food, those that are more yin tend to gravitate toward the periphery of the body, and the more yang foods gather at the center. In the kitchen, macrobiotic cooks try to retain as much of the vegetable as possible, in order to bring all its yin and all its yang qualities to the dish; carrots are never peeled, just washed, and their feathery tops are included in the dish or made into a condiment. The roots of leeks and scallions are cooked and eaten. If the universe is creating a wonderful, energized, whole vegetable, it only makes sense that we should eat as much of it as possible to receive its entire charge.

EXERCISE YOUR INNER COMPASS

Check out the trunk of a tree. It is gathered, tight, and compact (yang). From this gathered center, branches can push outward (yin), allowing for green leaves (mostly yin) to extend, creating the periphery. Here we see that yin and yang are truly antagonistic (completely opposite in their direction) and yet complementary; without the trunk, there can be no leaves, and without the leaves bringing nutrients from the sun, the trunk would eventually die.

When you're cutting vegetables for dinner, check out the centers and peripheries of all the natural foods you prepare.

law #8: there is nothing neutral: there is always yin or yang in excess

With respect to cooking and health, this law means that everything has some sort of impact. There is no neutral, free food, as we all thought popcorn was in our dieting days. Even water has a strong impact on the body. Everything has a charge, either more yin or more yang, and therefore every single element that you introduce into your cooking shifts the energy somehow.

In conventional weight-loss diets, calories are the yardstick of impact; the more calories you eat, the more weight you gain, right? But a 100-calorie dessert and 100 calories of salty pickle have completely different impacts on the body: one more yin and the other more yang. Foods that are more yin produce relaxation, expansion, talkiness, and, in the extreme, weakness or the softness of fatty weight gain. More yang foods create more active energy, tightness, and, in the extreme, rigidity. *Every* food has an energy charge. By keeping our food choices in the healthy, natural zone, we get to experience good-quality yinness and good-quality yangness, which keep our lives strong, flexible, and balanced. Health food may have had the reputation in the past as boring, dull, and sort of . . . neutral, but it ain't.

EXERCISE YOUR INNER COMPASS

Pull a vegetable from the fridge and get out a whole grain. Checking out the vegetable first, note its yinness and yangness. Now begin to make a judgment about which force dominates the other; is it more contracted than expanded, more hard than soft, more rigid than flowing? Which force would you say predominates in the vegetable? Which force is it "governed" by? Now look at the grain, and notice its qualities: Is it more yin or more yang?

Next, compare the vegetable and the grain: in terms of expansion and contraction, it is clear that the grain is more contracted, dry, and compact (yang) and that the vegetable is more expanded and moist (yin). The differences between these two foods make them a very dynamic pair of antagonistic, complementary opposites. Together, they produce a wonderful electricity that the body really grooves on.

law #9: yin and yang combined in varying proportions produce different phenomena. the attraction and repulsion among phenomena are proportional to the difference of the yin and yang forces

Macrobiotics is a comparison game. Nothing is completely yin; it is just more yin than something else. Perhaps it is less yin than another thing, in which case it may even start to look sort of . . . yang.

The degree to which something is yin or yang determines what it attracts and repels. When something is extremely yang, it attracts extreme yin. Moderate yin attracts moderate yang. Imagine a seesaw. The only thing to keep a kid at one end of the seesaw balanced is an equally weighted kid on the other end. When we pull either kid closer to the middle—without the other—balance is lost. But it's all a matter of proportion.

Ever eaten a steak and felt that you *must* have a beer with it or dessert right after? That is an example of very strong attraction between the steak (yang) and the dessert or alcohol (yin). That "must" is the stuff of compulsion, and the more we play with the extremes, the more we feel pushed around by forces beyond our control. Yin and yang are having their way with us. But after eating some barley, I don't feel that I *must* have a carrot, as though life just won't be right until I get that orange sucker inside of me. It might be nice to have some vegetables, but not necessary. This is because the yin-to-yang ratio between the grain and the vegetable is such that the seesaw of yin and yang is not being tilted much. I am just one inch from center eating grains, and one inch from center eating vegetables. Whereas a candy bar and a corned-beef sandwich will keep me teeter-tottering all day.

Another extremely important aspect of this law is that when the yinness or yangness of one thing changes, the degrees of attraction and repulsion change within the system, thereby affecting the whole. For example, if you change your behavior, how does it affect your relationships? Ever been in a relationship where you think, "I'm not usually like this." Maybe you generally talk a lot, but with one particular individual, you just listen. Or with one special person, you do lots and lots of talking. Someone who is very yin will bring out the yang in you, and vice versa. Standing next to an exceptionally beautiful person can make you feel ugly, and being near a not-so-good-looking person can make you feel like a beauty queen. Everything's relative, and each relationship has its own special charge, based upon the yin and yang forces within it.

If you change your behavior, how does it affect your family? If your sibling were to become a heroin addict, what impact would it have on the system? Who would be attracted to help her and who would be repelled? Who would become stronger, and who would be weakened by it?

The body is also a system, and what we do to it creates systemic change. Many modern medications change the presenting symptom, but, in so doing, they create a new imbalance elsewhere. We've all heard of the vicious cycle that the elderly can get into when pill number one helps with the arthritis but creates anxiety; pill number two helps with the anxiety but creates acid reflux, etc.

* * *

Millions of people are now taking an aspirin every day to prevent a heart attack, but what other systems are being thrown out of whack by that daily change? We weren't born with a bottle of aspirin in our hands, and if it is strong enough to thin the blood, it's gotta be strong enough to do other things. So let's ask ourselves: what do you think happens to contracted organs when they are subjected to strong expansion over time? How do you suppose expanded organs respond to excess expansion over time? Follow your intuition. Now let's look for the cause: if strong yin (aspirin) is the cure, then strong yang (constriction, thickening, hardening) must be the problem needing to be balanced. The macrobiotic mind asks the following question: what is causing the extreme yang condition in the first place? What are the yang factors that could be doing this? Animal food? Salt? Pressure and stress? Inherited belief systems? Lack of (yin) oxygen? The macrobiotic mind then looks to reduce the extreme yang factors (beginning with food), replacing them with better quality choices. By treating the symptom, we continue to create new imbalances. But by searching out and treating the cause, which is always some underlying imbalance in the yin-to-yang ratio, we can bring the system back to its original, dynamic natural template.

The more extreme the yin and yang components are, the stronger the energy between them. Hopefully, you are sensing the yinness and yangness of certain things and the charge that is created within that difference. At first, this may happen conceptually but it soon occurs intuitively. By working from your inner compass and understanding the laws of change, it is possible to heal yourself and live a life of ridiculous freedom.

EXERCISE YOUR INNER COMPASS

This is about sensing the energies between different things. Let's do a little exercise: go out and get an apple. And a saltine cracker. Put them next to each other and just relax. Let your inner compass feel if there is any relationship between them. If your mind chatters, don't worry. It doesn't matter. Just breathe and see what comes. Sense how they relate. Now take away the saltine and put a glass of water next to the apple. What has changed? Remove the apple and place a piece of bread next to the water. What do you feel? Take away the water and put a second slice of bread next to the first. What are you noticing? Subtle differences? No differences? Big ones?

· Rice Break ·

Notes from a three-day rice fast:

●   ●   ●

Day One: Uh . . . I feel stuck inside. Nothing is coming out. My personality has gone away somewhere, and I can't find it. I go to the computer to write, feel mentally constipated, and then turn away from the keyboard, staring at the desk.

I am being contracted by the rice, my core squeezed down to a yin-to-yang ratio of about 7 to 1. I am shutting down a bit as my body adjusts. Not the Chatty Cathy you are used to.

George Ohsawa suggested a ten-day rice fast for one purpose: spiritual growth. It is to bring me straight to my energetic center—which is like a radio antenna and transmitter—turning down the volume on the energy functioning at all other levels. This is not a place from which to live a normal life. This diet is for meditation.

I have read the above paragraphs five times now. I honestly can't tell if they are good or bad, catchy or boring. They simply are.

Uh-oh. Here we go. Critical judgment gone. Just being.

Not that I am wigging out. When others enter the room, interrupting what I'm doing, I interact with them very well. They have no idea that I am just the transmitter today, no longer editorializing, generating resentments, or . . . even thoughts. And I am nice. I am . . . rice. Endlessly patient, actually—I even stun myself, explaining something in more detail than I need to, or calmly giving way to someone in a hurry. Their hurry seems so strange to me. I couldn't hurry if I tried.

I AM SO IN-THE-MOMENT! I just sit here and breathe, trusting that something will come out of me, although each train of thought seems to have only two or three cars! When George Ohsawa did this diet, he would eat only brown rice and drink only twig tea for ten days. I don't know how he could do it. Day one is proving weird enough.

●   ●   ●

A memory bubble pops:

An ex-boyfriend of mine named Howard did this diet once for ten days when we were in New Mexico. I started it with him but could only handle three days because so many feelings came up, so much pain I had been repressing, that, on the third afternoon, I had to buy some carrot juice and an oatmeal cookie to shut up all the truth that was flying around inside of me. I didn't feel ready to go the desludging distance.

The boyfriend, however, persevered. One day we went to a very chi-chi spa outside of Santa Fe called Ten Thousand Waves, where we got delicious massages side by side from the most skilled and expensive hands. In the afternoon, we rented a private open-air hot tub and were bubbling away in very steamy wa-ter, right in the middle of the desert. The sky was crystal clear, a cool breeze blowing against my face as I relaxed, naked, in the tub. Howard, at this point, had been eating rice for seven days straight. He had been squeezed so hard that he looked lean and sinewy, his skin taut and glowing. He sat across from me in our private buck-a-minute bath, and it seemed, in my mind, like a decent time to fool around a little. Of course, this was just another way for me to hide out on my true feelings, but I was prepared to go for it. What the hell! No one was watching—I slithered toward him with a "come hither" grin.

Unfortunately, I had forgotten that I was dealing with RICE GUY. Having discharged so much energy sludge in the last week, his radio antenna was crys-tal clear and he was completely tuned in to my game. He could feel my mixed signals, my neurotic confusion, and my horniness as a cover. He could sense, by being so close to his truth, just how far I was from mine. My "Hey, let's get our two hundred bucks' worth out of this experience" rang within him as the cheap thought that it was. Not to mention that seven days of brown rice is not exactly an aphrodisiac. My slinky moves toward him were greeted with disdain and my kissy-face posturing rebuffed. I felt hurt, pissed off, and caught.

I remember thinking, in that moment, "A rice fast is not good for human relationships." And that wasn't just about my being confused and miserable. Ohsawa's ten-day rice fast is about connecting with the Infinite Universe, with which we have our primary relationship. The concept of energy pouring in at the head and down through the body begins to make actual sense when you're vibrating at 7 to 1. Eating only whole grain hooks you up to your intuition and the natural world with such incredible immediacy and clarity that it lends itself to small-talky human interaction the way taking a hit of acid lends itself to a board meeting.

And that's why, in everyday life, I eat more than just rice. Vegetables, beans, fish, fruit, and other good-quality foods give me a little more oomph, and the flexibility needed to move laterally in this world. I don't want to be hooked up vertically like a monk all the time. I want to watch old movies and write books and mope on the couch when he doesn't call. I want to be greedy and take big risks, sometimes winning, sometimes losing, so that I can feel proud or battered and then I will crawl home again, to 7 to 1, where I see that it's all just a game.

That's why, if I were to distill this book down to one sentence, it would be:

EAT WHOLE GRAINS. They build this home inside. They provide the relationship with the Infinite Universe in spite of the chocolate fudge sundae you dollop on top. With grains in the middle, life becomes the spokes radiating out from the steady, solid wheel rolling us through existence.

Uh-oh. I'm becoming RADIO ANTENNA gal now. I just went into the kitchen to talk to my mother, and I simply responded to her. No neurotic energy bomb to lob onto the scene, no funny thought motivating me to get giggly and stupid, I just stared and smiled. I'm RICE GAL now, pleasant enough, just getting more rice and some tea, thank you very much. Leaving kitchen now.

I can't force anything from this state. All I can do, when I'm feeling at a loss for words, is sit back, relax, trust that my transmitter is tuned in to the big cosmic radio station, and wait. If the Infinite Universe wants me to say something, it'll come. It makes me understand why Japanese art is so spare. Haikus so tidy. The more I press for product, the less I get. The rice produces automatic surrender.

Every sound is coming in loud and clear. My fingers hitting the keyboard are like a funny, tribal beat. The computer's hum is louder than usual. Normally the noise in my head would push these things into the background, but the head noise is gone. Every sound pipes up to express itself, from the creaking of my chair to the ticking of a clock, to my squealing nephews in the other room. Even the swallowing of my tea presents itself in Dolby Surround Sound. But it is all pleasant. The antenna is clear today.

Stringing thoughts together seems like an intellectual game, or the crocheting of a rug—just for fun. I'm going to stop writing now. Nothing's coming. See you tomorrow.

·   ·   ·

Day Two: I am feeling rather fresh and perky. I have already noticed that my body is changing—skin smoother, I feel lighter and leaner. My body is becoming more yang, which means energy is pulling in toward the center of my being. Excess yin, in the form of fluids and acids, is being discharged, leaving my body feeling balanced and light. When I move, I feel as though I am animated from my skeleton, as opposed to my muscles. It's as if I am a marionette, with the strings being pulled from somewhere above me. I call it the "Fred Astaire" feeling.

I am in Cornwall as I write. It is the land of English romance novels: rolling hills, thatched-roof cottages, and sheep roaming behind little stone walls. My mother, now a great macro cook, lives here with her husband, and I try to come and visit at least once a year. Their apartment, very cozy and inviting, is perched on a hill right on the bank of a tidal river. From every window of the apartment, I can see water flowing up the river to the town of Truro. When the tide recedes, it flows back out to sea. Sometimes the river is full like a bathtub, and sometimes the river is nothing more than a trickle between two smelly mudflats. Yin and yang.

My mother lives in a tiny village of about 160 people. From here, one can walk over a big hill and through a farm to another tiny town called St. Clements. This little hike, to and from my mother's house, takes about an hour. It requires big rubber boots to handle the mud of the path and a penchant for cows, who will be found grazing somewhere on the hill. Normally, when I consider walking to St. Clements, I feel slightly ambivalent. It's really not a hard walk, "but there is that big hill and . . . I dunno. Maybe later. Oh, shoot. Come on." There is a tug-of-war between the cells in my body aching to go and the ones that are committed to the couch. I generally end up going (feeling too much like a loser if I don't), but the argument does take place.

This morning was different. All that was required to make the trip to St. Clements was the mental casting out of my mind, as light as a fishing line, over to the little village. I set it, mentally, as the goal. Done. With the goal hooked into the little stone church on the other side of the hill, my body responded. No stress. No arguments. My legs felt light, yet strong and enthusiastic, about the trek. They simply followed the order my mind had issued. It was as if my mind, locked in the St. Clements church, was reeling my body over the hill like a (happy) fish.

Meanwhile, another part of my mind, the part that receives and enjoys sensation, was walking with me. Acutely aware of the damp leaves, the gnarled roots, and the fresh mud on the path, I enjoyed the walk from a freakily still place within myself. Normally, this trek becomes a walking meditation that allows my mind simply to wander off, solving problems, generating fantasies, etc. This time, my mind stayed centered in my body, getting off on the scents in the air, the mysterious, mystical copse of Harry Potterish pines in the middle of the hike, and the curious looks on the faces of the cows.

These are the moments of which, upon our deathbeds, I think we'll all wish we'd had more. When the body and mind have slowed down enough simply to receive, we are truly in our lives; we see, for the first time, the funny wrinkle on our lover's face. We feel the silky skin of the four-year-old's hand. We detect a taste in our favorite food we'd never noticed before. Some people spend years practicing mediation or yoga or t'ai chi to get themselves to slow down to this place, but they are constantly fighting the speediness of the food they are ingesting. Just eat brown rice for a day. Chew it well.

These moments, timeless, thoughtless diamonds of perception, are the ones that get recorded, deep within the subconscious mind, so that when we want to relive them, through meditation or hypnosis, or in our dreams, they are there, springing forth with their original intensity.

Uh-oh. I'm getting silly now. It's afternoon number two and I am dancing around the kitchen like Muhammad Ali, punching the air, fake-punching my mother. I squeeze her face, calling her "Little Susie," which, because of her big cheeks, causes me to giggle uncontrollably like the stoner I once was. Pure energy is shooting out of me. Ripples of power emanating from my body. I want to jump around for hours. Instead of standing still, I move from side to side, hopping on the balls of my feet, driving everyone around me nuts. I miss other foods today, feeling a twinge of self-pity about the couscous cake my mother is making, but I know I will get some on Monday when I go back to the sludgy, sensory-driven being that I usually am. Right now, I am RICE GAL! Look out!

Yin and yang make perfect sense to me now. Organic, living things seem more compelling than man-made things. I sense their centers and their peripheries, their vital energy and the changeability within them. I notice if something is more expanded or contracting, dry or wet. I feel that I'm viewing the world through the lens of a hallucinogenic; I am seeing the spirals in things.

* * *

Day Three: THIS SUCKS. Because the rice has me so in-the-moment, I wasn't sure I could stand another freakin' second of it as I embarked on my meditation this morning. I just needed a break, for cryin' out loud, from the stillness, the slowness, and the seriousness of it all. Hence, I embarked on a full-blown fantasy about Michael coming back, basically un-dumping me, followed by my cool and oh-so-satisfying response to his entreaties.

But it was weird. In a normal fantasy, my mental energy has a tendency to spin off, morphing like a dream, into other themes. People's faces are fuzzy, re-actions unclear, or only flash for a split second, until it all tumbles into a differ-ent color, grocery store, or bed. My challenge is to keep it reeled in.

This morning, I had the opposite problem; stuff stayed still. He was clear, I was clear, I could even picture his face like a photograph. He pulled me over to a secluded corner of the restaurant and told me how much he missed me. I could hear his voice, how he would say every word, and the nervous little man-nerisms that would come between movements of the conversation. As he drew closer, the unique chemistry of our chakras came back to me, stirring my whole body. There is something so amazing about chemistry, how we make a unique perfume with every person. And sometimes we can chase that particular scent forever.

But it was all such hard work! My mind didn't want to budge. The rice is strong and proud and so sticky they use it on the back of Chinese postage stamps. But I persevered. As I slid these crystalline blocks together, one by one, re-creating our personal universe like an ice sculpture, I assumed it would get all sexy at one point. But no. The rice kept me chaste. The rice is a monk. No wonder Howard gave me the hot-tub rebuff! Rice would not give me the oomph, the sweat, the excitement of a roll in the mental hay. My body will not generate the hormones right now. Frustrated, feeling like "What the hell is wrong with me?" I suddenly remember that for the last sixty hours, all I have put in my body is rice. I slap myself (gently) on the forehead. One purpose: spir-itual development.

I don't want to live from this place for too long; I miss my mother's macro cooking, and I enjoy writing much more when I'm a tiny bit sludgy. But like trying that new drug in college, I'm glad I did it once. I feel as though I am coming from a completely different place inside myself—a place I didn't even know was there. It's as if I have meditated for three years, and all I did was chew some bowls of rice. My personality has undergone a refreshing pruning. I feel young and flexible. In the mirror, my eyes look sparkly and mischievous, as they gaze—like a wise old soul inside a newborn baby—upon the invisible.

laws 10, 11, and 12

The following laws are my favorites, for they pose the greatest challenges to linear, logical Western thinking. By accepting that "yin changes into yang" and "yang changes into yin," the real fun begins. In this chapter, we look closely at seasonal change as an example of everything eventually becoming its opposite. But that's just the beginning: every natural phenomenon, including the wonderful mystery of a love affair, follows these distinct laws of change. Now that you've studied yin and yang quite closely, you're ready for the mind-blowing stuff. Hang on and enjoy the ride!

law #10: all phenomena are ephemeral, constantly changing their constitution of yin and yang forces; yin changes into yang, yang changes into yin

and

law #11: extreme yin produces yang, and extreme yang produces yin

We already understand that, because the universe produces endless change, nothing stays the same over time. But this principle is saying that, as stuff changes, it is not completely random in its metamorphosis. When witnessed over the very long run, it becomes clear that yang things are becoming yin and yin things are becoming yang. Just hang out in nature for a little while, and this restlessness reveals itself. Within our lifetimes, we go from a tight, compact spiral in our mother's womb to a big, tall, fully expressed adult. Later, we contract again, shrinking and shriveling with age. Flowers bloom and die. Even hard rocks become loose sand over time.

The most obvious example of this journey from yin to yang is seasonal change. Within the span of a year, we—especially in the temperate zone—experience incredible, miraculous movements between opposites that, if we examine them closely, are our greatest teachers.

But this shifting between yin and yang occurs on every level; businesses experience their vicissitudes, as do countries. Perhaps most compelling are the shifts we experience in intimate relationships. A love relationship is a spiral, with two people going over the same material—each other—over and over again, but with a deeper and stronger appreciation of the partner every time. Although these changes do not necessarily occur when the seasons change—and each partner may experience them at different times—our emotional cycles go from yin to yang just like everything else.

THE FIVE TRANSFORMATIONS OF ENERGY

In Eastern thinking, there exist five distinct transformations of energy in the cycle between yin and yang. These same transformations are identified as the seasons (which include a fifth season, late summer). In this chapter, we will look at qualities of each energy transformation, the season it creates, and how we cook to harmonize with it. Finally, we'll look at what happens when we experience these transformations in intimacy.

Spring

In the springtime, we experience upward, rising energy. Daffodils, tulips, all the first flowers of spring are dominated by this powerful, upward surge. Spirits "lift" in the spring, and the religious symbols all bring us to the idea of renewed life, or rebirth. The wind picks up and the air is clear as the earth is swept by refreshing, renewing force. We all come out of the house and feel like jumping for

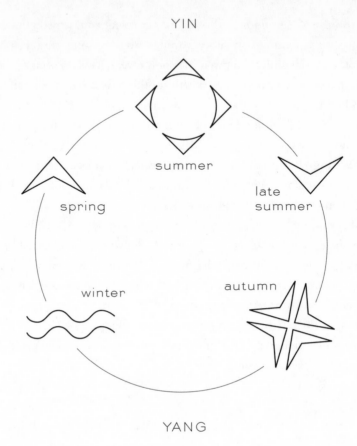

YIN

summer

late
summer

spring

autumn

winter

YANG

joy, also an expression of the yin energy we are actually feeling throughout our bodies. This is a time to clean the house or go on a fast in order to eliminate winter's possible stagnation and make room for the lighter vibes of spring.

We naturally lighten up our eating in the spring—less oil and quicker cooking styles, in order to let the strong upward energy express itself. We are attracted to fresh, green, upward-growing foods and light grains like barley and wheat. The liver, the vital organ most governed by upward energy, receives a strong dose of natural, upward vibes in the spring, as does its partner, the gall bladder. A stuffy liver makes you irritable and cranky. A clear and healthy liver supports patience and creativity.

Love relationships usually begin with a nice dose of upward energy. This is the lovely springtime of love. You are fresh and new to each other, and you feel a huge "lift" in each other's presence. Sexual attraction and sensitivity are high, and the thrill of it all can feel as if your head is being blown off from all the upward, rising force.

Summer

As upward energy reaches its peak, it expands outward; this is the active, plasmic energy transformation we call summer. The blooms of summer are luscious and juicy compared to the polite and delicate buds of spring. Everything is big, open, and expanded. Warm weather causes us to slow down, rolling down the beaches in a lazy, relaxed way as opposed to the cheery clip of spring. Parties take place outside, and everyone seems to travel somewhere, both expressions of expansive forces. The earth pushes out an incredible abundance of fruits and vegetables, juicy and full. Consciousness is generally outward—allowing us to "come out" of ourselves, not so hypnotized by our inner worlds. Rushes of expansive energy through the body produce feelings of joy and contentment. People feel passionately about summer because it is the season of fire. The incredible warm, active vibes of summer cause the expansion of our bodies and spirits.

In the summer, we cook with a higher, more intense flame in dishes like stirfries. Roasting and grilling are also popular in the summer, introducing the foods to strong doses of extreme, searing heat. Broad leafy greens, which have drunk in lots of sunshine and have a slightly bitter taste, are perfect for summer eating. Fruits and moist vegetables like cucumbers are luscious and necessary to cool the body. Corn, as a grain or vegetable, is yellow like the sun and imparts a sweet, expansive energy that charges the heart. Of your internal organs, it is the heart and small intestine that are most nourished by the expansive, plasmic energy of summer.

A healthy love relationship goes from its own spring to summer; attraction and euphoria become love. Your heart is strongly activated by fire energy, and you're both consumed by positive feelings for each other generated at the heart chakra. Thinking of your beloved literally "warms" your heart. You've talked and shared and laughed a lot, opening yourselves up, like blossoming flowers. A deep vibrational exchange is occurring, and your auras are beginning to balance each other. If you haven't bedded each other yet, it feels very natural to do so now.

Late Summer

We in the West don't identify this season officially, but it is the time from about August through September, sometimes referred to as Indian summer. As the transition from the fully expanded energy of summer into autumn takes place, the intensity lessens and the energy begins to settle. This is the pause before expansion becomes contraction. Lethargy overtakes us in this postcoital space-out of the year. It is no accident that many of the warmer cities of Europe basically shut down as the entire population goes on a monthlong vacation. As the energy drops, there begins a definite "settling in" feeling as school resumes and people begin to execute their plans for the fall.

Late summer is a sweet time, as the harvests come in and the warmth of the summer has settled into our bodies and consciousness. Round, sweet, balancing foods like onions and squash feel perfect for this mellow time of year, and as the weather subtly shifts to cool, cooking styles like slow steaming (*nishime*) impart a steady, warming vibe into food. Your stomach, spleen, and pancreas—major digestive organs—are nourished by the downward, settling energy of late summer, so sweet and settling foods like sweet rice and millet are the grains emphasized during this time of year.

In the downward and settling phase of a love relationship, the passion recedes a bit, which is normal because nothing can maintain peak intensity forever. If the couple has compatibility beyond attraction, they can "settle into" this phase of relating to each other. The intimacy explored in sex feels deeper now as they know each other better. The taste associated with this energy is sweet, and this phase of a relationship can feel very sweet and soothing.

Autumn

Thanksgiving is a great symbol of autumnal energy; a gathering of people, food, and emotions all represent this yang transformation of energy. As nature's force begins to pull in, we do, too. We become more introspective, addressing relationships and personal goals. Life feels a little more serious than it does in summer and can border on melancholic as the trees drop their leaves. The pulling in is taking place on all levels, within the body and without. This is the most yang time of the year.

Fall cooking is warm and intended to help energy move deep into the body, just as energy is pulling into the trees, and into the earth. More root vegetables, plus long, slow cooking and especially pressure-cooking do the job of driving energy deep into our bodies and strengthening our cores. Short-grain rice and a pungent taste are emphasized in the fall. Your lungs and large intestine are the organs most sensitive to—and nourished by—autumn's gathering energy, which can cause the lungs to discharge phlegm and fluid at this time of year.

In a relationship, at a certain point, each individual's energy will begin to gather in toward itself. The incredible explosion of outward energy, which is falling in love, must be tempered by attention to one's self, in order to integrate all the new information. As each partner pulls inside, individuation takes place so that, hopefully, this couple can strike the balance between being two people and one partnership—the ultimate paradox. The original upward energy has turned into its opposite. But that is simply the universe's pattern.

Winter

Imagine your winter coat. Gloves. Seeing your breath. Cold air on your cheeks. Our part of the planet has pulled away from the sun so it becomes extremely cold, which creates contraction. Everything is dark, and all the living things go inward. Trees have pulled their sap in and down. Bears hibernate. People go to indoor parties, huddling together for a type of warmth they don't even know they are seeking. The weather outside is extremely yin (cold, dark), and that produces a yang response in us; our bodies fight to stay warm, active, and gathered. We are literally floating in an in-between that eventually becomes the strong expansion of spring.

In winter we need to stay warm. More oil, hearty soups, animal food, and rich bean dishes are necessary in a five-season climate. Baking feels comforting. Even deep-frying is appropriate for sealing warmth into the body. Buckwheat, beans, sea vegetables, and good-quality salt are all very nourishing to the kidneys, bladder, and reproductive organs—those most strongly charged by winter's inward, floating energy.

In a relationship, this phase can scare people. The feelings of passion seem to go so deeply subterranean, it's as if they'd disappeared. Just as in winter, the energy is so still that it's hard to believe that upward energy will ever come again. Winter requires faith and patience, especially in a relationship. It is a good time to go inward and clean out your own emotional closet (through therapy, meditation, journaling, etc.), so that you are clear and generous when the upward and outward energy returns. Or it may be the perfect time to go deep into the relationship and work out any conflict or stagnation that has been left unaddressed between the two of you. This work will make room for the passionate, springtime energy to return easily and happily. If a relationship accrues great resentment, it is in the spring, when upward energy returns, that the resentment can come up and out with great force, exploding like a bomb. The relationship is receiving a spring cleaning from the Infinite Universe. Although we think of spring as the time when people get together, it is also the season of breakups.

BALANCING EXTREMES: CONTRACTION AND EXPANSION

In order to do this dance, you must have the strength to contract and the flexibility to expand. If contraction and expansion begin with forces yin and yang entering and exiting the earth, you should be receiving these forces easily and in the ratio most suited to human health. It is believed in macrobiotic theory that the human organism is created by a ratio of roughly 7 parts heaven's force to 1 part earth's force (yin). Of course, the ratio is slightly different for everyone, but it is believed that we live in that range. Therefore, the rice plant, which is more like 7 parts earth's force (yin) to 1 part heaven's (yang), provides great balance for the human body.

All whole grains have yin-to-yang ratios that harmonize with the human body. If you are feeling out of sorts, chew some rice or other grain to come back to center. Adding vegetables makes the yin-to-yang ratio a little wider and more relaxed, but still totally within a healthy range. You will find, as you become more sensitive, that each grain make you feel slightly different, so experiment and find out what works for you.

A candy bar, full of white sugar, creates an enormous amount of expansion for the human organism. Too much expansive energy, and you can become depressed, inactive, spaced-out, and may ultimately be prone to diseases like leukemia, schizophrenia, anemia, brain cancer, breast cancer, skin cancer, and any other condition governed by upward, outward, spreading energy. A sirloin steak, on the other hand, introduces excessively strong contraction to the human organism. With too much contracting energy, you can become tight, inflexible, and mentally rigid. Diseases that are the products of overcontraction include atherosclerosis (*sclerosis* means hardening), cardiac arrest, cervical cancer, bone cancer, and any other condition that is governed by downward, hardening, contracting energy.

But the strangest phenomenon of all, and the most challenging to the Western mind, is getting too much yin and too much yang at the same time. But, surely, that makes no sense: they cancel each other out, no? No. Too much yin and too much yang combined mean that the quality of expansive energy being introduced into the body is extreme compared to what the human organism needs and that the quality of contraction is also extreme compared to nature's template as well.

In fact, because yin and yang attract each other so strongly, it is very common that one extreme attracts the other. The body can sustain the extremes for a remarkably long time, but it is inevitable, if we continue to violate the rhythms and laws of nature, that our physical vehicles will suffer. You could win the energy lottery by getting a heart attack AND depression!

In terms of feelings and behavior, I have begun to expect things to turn into their opposite; if I am *madly* passionate about someone, I have the tendency to become angry and repulsed by him at some point. In the classes that I teach, it is the most skeptical participants who are the poster children for macrobiotics by the end of the course. The most dramatic stories of recovery from addiction come after the most pathetic, horrible despair. Where there is resistance, there is enormous positive energy lurking, and as long as I am patient, the change will come about. The universe is fundamentally alchemical by nature, and for us to expect mechanical, logical progressions to take place is utterly delusional. The more I recognize the laws of yin and yang, so magical and fluid, the more I can recognize these patterns and "play" in my own life.

As you develop your macrobiotic mind, you will see that everything is—slowly or quickly—turning into its opposite. Where has this principle played out in your life already? Did you ever strongly dislike someone only to discover later that he was a true friend? How many movies begin with the leading man and lady positively despising each other so that we can watch the transformation into love? Or the opposite: ever married for life and then ended up in a courtroom? What happened?

Moods are good examples of extremes becoming their opposites: after the explosion of a heated argument, you feel peaceful and strangely closer to the person you were fighting with. A good cry leads to laughter. The frisky, heated buildup of sexual tension climaxes and immediately becomes its opposite of deep relaxation, and sometimes even repulsion. You save your pennies for ten years to buy a home, only to suffer buyer's remorse a week later. Controlling parents inadvertently create little rebels.

But keep in mind that after yang becomes yin, it just becomes yang again. Your kid won't leave you alone one day, screeches that she hates you the next, only to draw you the most beautiful picture on the weekend, so we can never relax into thinking we have it all set.

The more we eat according to nature's laws, the better we can live with the universe's inevitable pattern of change. When we become very sludgy, either nature's process of change gets slowed down or it begins to create mutations and weird illnesses. When we look for life to stay still, to go in only one direction, or to be controllable, we have lost our freedom.

EXERCISING YOUR INNER COMPASS

The journey from yin to yang (or vice versa) is evident in food—hard carrots become soft; soft bread becomes hard. Fresh things become decayed, and smelly compost provides nutrients for new growth. Identify another example of radical change in the kitchen.

Now consider these questions: what changes do you witness on a daily basis? What, in your life, has turned into its opposite? What changes have you seen in politics? What kinds of shifts have you watched your parents go through over the long haul? If you have children or nephews and nieces, study them for radical shifts from one extreme to the other. Some things will be immediately evident, while others seem to defy this law. Be patient and allow your perspective to widen.

law #12: big yin attracts small yin, and big yang attracts small yang

I've kept this one till the end, just to confuse us thoroughly. When people eat lots and lots of yin all the time, they crave more yin. Someone who loves salty foods can crave more salt, as opposed to (or as well as) sugar. There is a point where an organism, when it is strongly charged in one direction, attracts not only its opposite but also more of its own. For instance, a guru or a cult attracts a follower. But a follower does not attract an organization. The army attracts more military-minded people. A family pulls its family members into itself. Like-minded people tend to congregate.

Ever notice that a baby always steals the attention in a room? We are hypnotized by this tight, compact, hot little spiral of joy, and all the adult attention is literally pulled toward the strong yang energy. Although a baby is smaller than an adult, its yang charge is greater and therefore is "big yang" in this equation.

When it comes to attraction between the sexes, men go crazy not only for all our estrogen but *that* little sachet of testosterone we carry around inside of us which drives them over the edge with desire. Big testosterone attracting little testosterone. Likewise, women always go sniffing around for that hidden softness inside every tough guy, and it is our big femaleness that brings it out in them. Relationships are complex, healing, and balancing mechanisms . . . but more on that later.

Nature is a great example of big yin—it is expansive, flexible, and varied. Most people are attracted to nature because it brings out some of those qualities in ourselves. In the great outdoors, our spirits (small yin) feel expanded and unfettered. Those, however, who are cut off from their spirits don't let that energy flow, and they seek to dominate nature with their brute force. Luckily, nature bats last.

EXERCISING YOUR INNER COMPASS

Where are you attracted to similarity? Which organizations do you belong to?
How does an organization bring out certain qualities or strengths in you? How
does adult peer pressure operate in your life?

part two

becoming a macro chick

Welcome to the next stop on your adventure. Having learned so much about the order of the universe, you are armed with a new pair of glasses through which to see the world. So put on your yin/yang specs as we look at food and the role it will play in your life as a healthy, beautiful, tuned-in macro chick!

phase one: going with the grain

G rain is the superfood. The überfood. The king. Grain rules. All you need to do to begin improving your life on all levels is to make whole grain a regular daily food. As the principal food in the macrobiotic diet, you should get to know whole grain—intimately. This is Phase One.

let's make it official

I would like to suggest that, in order to get the greatest results from this experiment, you eat whole grains at one meal (two if possible) each day for the next thirty days. You don't have to cook every day; most dishes last two or three days. Mix things up by alternating between plain grain and fancy grain dishes. Once a day, chew your grain really well—like fifty times a mouthful. If that's too hard, start lower, but aim for fifty, and then one hundred when you've reached that. If you can, make some time to eat alone, so you can really relax and chew. We need to get this wonderful stuff in you and have you begin to absorb it well.

Within thirty days, you should notice some changes. Your mind may feel clearer after chewing well. Perhaps your body's daily discharges will feel different. You may become less interested in some foods and more interested in others. Regardless of what you register consciously, whole grains are feeding you—pumping minerals, vitamins, fiber, and the amazing, balancing vibes of the natural universe into your body. They are a force to be reckoned with. Give them a chance.

You may want to stay in Phase One for two months, or three, or even a year. It doesn't matter. Just chew grain and see how you feel. Unless you suffer from a particular allergy or intolerance, you cannot go wrong with grain.

In this chapter, I have included a bunch of whole-grain recipes so you can dive into cooking right now. Just eat the way you normally do, adding these powerful little suckers to the mix. Although you will get more dramatic results if you actually replace your old carbs like white rice, white bread, white noodles, and potatoes with whole grains, that's not absolutely necessary at this point. Macrobiotics is about experimenting and discovering how things work for you. Take it at your own pace. If you want to dive in a little deeper right now, go to the recipes later in the book, and feel free to use any of them now to complement your grain dishes.

WHOLE GRAIN IS CIVILIZED

Modern civilization was born with the active cultivation of grain. It is believed that we went from generally nomadic peoples to an agricultural type when we realized how incredibly cool grain was. With this discovery came the planting of row after row of peaceful, graceful grain, each stalk yielding thousands of seeds for every one planted. Suddenly, there was incredible abundance—grain to eat, grain to trade, grain to store, and enough left over to throw at weddings! Like Microsoft in the eighties, grain is an excellent investment with mind-blowing returns.

WHOLE GRAIN IS GOOD FOR YOUR BRAIN

So the cultivation of grain settled us, at least for the period until harvesting, and in that time, we began to think. You see, grain is energy food, and it is especially supportive of sustained mental energy, since its complex carbohydrates, broken down by chewing, create a peaceful, steady rise in blood sugar to the brain.

a word about carbohydrates

The most recent trend in eating is high-protein, low-carbohydrate diets. The theory goes that by abstaining from carbohydrates—the fuel that the body needs for energy—stored fat begins to convert itself into useable glucose. Therefore, you lose weight. Sounds good.

However, when considering food, we need to look beyond our bikinis at the overall picture. You are a human with a physical self, an emotional being, creativity, intellect, relationships, and a spiritual life. All these aspects of who you are get nourished (or malnourished) by the foods that you eat. Although Dr. Atkins hit the nail on the head by identifying simple carbohydrates like sugar and white flour as sources of useless empty calories, his plan never fully appreciates the benefits of complex carbohydrates and, specifically, whole grains. Whole grains feed your spirit, mind, and body while helping you to cultivate emotional and energetic integrity; they make you whole. Lifelong issues and problems can get healed by eating whole grains over a period of months or years. A hunk of pig muscle delivers something completely different. Plus, whole grains do not raise the blood sugar in such a violent way as to bring on an assault of insulin, which Dr. Atkins blames for obesity.

Although, by eating lots of meat, eggs, and cream all day, you may be losing some weight (in the short run), you are simultaneously starving yourself of the fuel that runs your humanity. One could even argue—if one tended toward the groovy and philosophical—that you are, by concentrating almost exclusively on animal food and animal products, getting intimate with our four-legged friends in a way that's de-evolutionary; we wonder why violence, materialism, and predatory behavior are out of control? We wonder why we treat one another like animals? Look at what we're eating!

And finally, because the human body needs carbohydrates, extremely low-carb diets may be a long and sexy setups for binges on sweets, bread, or alcohol. We need carbohydrates to function. They are our natural fuel. It is the quality of the carbs that is key, and whole grains are nicely balanced for the human body. Macrobiotic eating does not create thin, healthy bodies because you are starving yourself of nourishment and going into ketosis, complete with bad breath and constipation. Rather, as you eat plant-quality, whole, and fibrous foods packed with minerals, vitamins, and energy, you blossom like the beautiful, graceful, multipetaled flower that you are.

WHOLE GRAIN IS SOCIAL FOOD

Observe a field of wheat. Every stalk stands completely strong and independent, reaching unabashedly toward the heavens. Meanwhile, the plants are able to grow very close together, never strangling or crowding one another. The stalks bend and dance in a graceful group, like a school of fish or a flock of birds that thinks as a whole. In all cultures, one shares a meal (in fact, the word *meal* means grain) in order to connect deeply with a neighbor. It's no accident that we refer to this coming together as "breaking bread."

WHOLE GRAIN IS GROOVY

Eating grain brings about holistic thinking, without effort. How long have you been meditating, doing yoga, or praying in order to love your neighbor? Is it working? What charities to do support in order to forge a connection to the world? All that is great, but just chew whole grains extremely well every day and you will automatically begin to feel that deep connection to the rest of humanity you have been looking for. Whole grains are the perfect food for juggling the paradox of self and community and can lead to very trippy thinking. Imparting smooth, peaceful, strong energy, grains will keep you groovy over the long haul.

WHOLE GRAIN IS CHEAP

Organic brown rice costs about ninety cents a pound. Millet is even cheaper. It's just as well savvy businessmen don't know how amazing whole grain is, because given its actual value, they'd jack it up to a thousand bucks an ounce. Whole grain is also very cheap to grow, compared to feeding, protecting, and slaughtering animals.

WHOLE GRAIN IS STRONG

Put a banana on the kitchen counter and see how long it lasts before decay sets in. Try a steak. Now a glass of milk. These foods begin to stink, break down, and die within a week. Now put a grain of brown rice on the counter. Watch it closely for decay. Keep watching. If all you did were to watch that little grain, you'd lose your job, alienate your family, and starve to death a hundred times over before that little grain showed any sign of decomposition. Kept in its hull, it can stay strong and useable for THOUSANDS of years. Out of the hull, it will lose some of its energy but will be eaten by smart little critters long before it actually deteriorates on its own. In the absence of pests, it will last for years.

MEET THE FAMILY

We are lucky to have so many grains. Each one has a different personality and a unique energetic impact on the body. Grains, as a group, are the closest things to nutritionally complete food for human beings, containing amino acids, carbohydrates, fiber, minerals, vitamins, and fat. Because most of our ancestors were built on grain, we actually have a genetic relationship to the stuff, and our bodies respond quickly and happily to whole grain, the way a baby responds to mother's milk. Grain will create lasting endurance, calm in the face of adversity, and intuition at exactly the right moment. It will glow from inside of you, lightening not only your step but also your general vibe in the world. It will strengthen and heal your internal organs and then move on to alter your thoughts. It will give you the ability to do things you never thought possible. This book was written by whole grains.

Rice

There are many types of rice: long grain, medium grain, short grain, and basmati, for a start. The longer the grain, the more relaxing the rice is, so long is used mostly in summer, short in fall and winter. Medium is used here and there.

Rice creates very strong gathering energy and is therefore a tonic to the lungs and large intestines, organs that gather wastes and release them. Considered particularly good for spiritual pursuits, rice strikes a balance between minerals, protein, and carbohydrates in such a way that it mirrors nature's energies beautifully. My only complaint about rice is that, in macrobiotics, it can sometimes be considered the *perfect* grain, and so I have seen lots of people basically OD on it. Too much rice is too much gathering energy. We need variety throughout the energy spectrum, as you shall see later on. So be sure to eat lots of different grains. Don't get stuck on rice.

Barley

I love barley, for its energy as much as its taste. Barley is upward, unsticky, and loose. It's a tonic to the liver and very good for the skin. Cooling and relaxing, barley is especially good cooked with rice or in soups. When cooking barley, be sure to use hulled barley—as opposed to pearled—because its minerals and fibers remain intact.

Buckwheat

Buckwheat, a native of Russia and China, is intense. Buckwheat is so warming and strengthening and absorbs so much fluid that, if eaten too often, it can create tightness and dryness in the body. Used occasionally in salads with sautéed vegetables, buckwheat is particularly good for the kidneys, bladder, and reproductive organs.

Millet

High in protein and fat and slightly alkaline, millet has served as a dietary staple of China, India, Egypt, and Northern Africa. Too bad we in the United States associate it with bird food. Millet is a tonic to the stomach, spleen, and pancreas, has a very centering and soothing effect on the body, and is great for making patties, burgers, or soups.

Oats

Yum. Who doesn't like oats already? They are sweet, creamy, and very satisfying. They also happen to be extremely high in protein, minerals, and vitamins B and E. In macrobiotic cooking, we try to use whole oats in order to benefit from the whole energy of the food, but steel-cut or rolled oats show up now and then. Oats grow best in cool, moist climates, making them a historic favorite in northern parts of Europe. Horses like them, too.

Quinoa (pronounced *Keen-wah*)

Grown originally in the high Andes of South America, quinoa is part of what made Incan civilization so incredible. It is now cultivated on other continents, and in different climates, proving its strength and adaptability. Because of the harsh circumstances under which it developed—high winds, strong sun, cold nights—quinoa has become very hardy, and one of its protective mechanisms is a coating of a bitter substance called saponin (which protects it from strong sunlight and needs to be rinsed off before cooking). Quinoa is one of the best sources of protein in the plant world. Its cousin, also native to the Andes, is an even smaller grain called amaranth. Quinoa is great cooked with rice or on its own. It can be the base for wonderful summer salads or cooked with extra water to make a porridge or soup—big hits in Peru!

Wheat

Wheat has been North America's darling grain since it was introduced in the early seventeenth century and has been cultivated for roughly ten thousand years. It was the Egyptians who discovered that wheat had enough gluten to be made into leavened bread. Since then, it has proven itself to be a most versatile and convenient food. However, since it is used mostly as a refined flour product these days, lots of people suffer allergies to wheat due to overrefining, rancid flour, and overconsumption. Macrobiotic cooking uses whole-wheat flour products but also the whole-wheat berry itself, usually cooked with rice. There may not be an allergic reaction to the whole grain.

Spelt

Wheat's cousin, spelt goes back to Southeast Asia from whence it was brought to Europe via the Middle East. Spelt-flour products are currently in vogue because people who are allergic to wheat tend to be able to tolerate spelt, which can be made into bread and noodles. A long grain, with a hard and thick husk, spelt is considered very tough, hearty, and good for overall immunity.

Rye

Generally used for hearty rye bread, this hard little grain is delicious soaked and then cooked with rice. Excellent for the liver, and reducing plaques in the body, rye has a rich and hearty European history as wonderful as the grain itself.

Corn

The corn used by the Native Americans was a heartier, dried version known as dent corn, which was always cooked with lime. Corn, very low in niacin, needed lime to balance its deficiencies. Polenta and cornmeal, which require no balancing if a variety of other grains is being eaten, are the versions used most in macrobiotic cooking. Corn's energy is particularly nourishing to the heart and small intestine.

Hato Mugi

Actually a grass, this food (also known as Job's Tears and pearl—as opposed to pearled—barley) has been a hit in China for four thousand years. Whole hato mugi comes in small, round balls with a beige husk, but very often only the polished, huskless version is available. Hato mugi is great in soups, stews, grain salads, or cooked with rice. Light, delicious, and wonderful for the skin, Hato mugi is one of my favorite foods.

Teff

You know you're really macro when you go to the trouble of finding teff. The tiniest grain there is, teff is the staple food of Ethiopia, a nation that has never been conquered by an outside people. Generally used for injera bread, teff also makes a nice porridge. It is high in calcium and other minerals.

SOAKING GRAINS

Spelt, rye, wheat berries, whole oats, and wild rice all need to be soaked in spring water for a few hours (but preferably overnight) before cooking. Otherwise, they end up chewy and hard to digest. Some people also soak their barley, hato mugi, and rice (quinoa, millet, and buckwheat are more often roasted). In general, soaking the above grains makes them more digestible and reduces any acidity that they may produce. Soaking is all the rage in macrobiotics these days and is a very good habit to get into.

COMBINING GRAINS

The recipes beginning on page 83 are fancy and delicious—most contain strong seasonings, fruit, or yummy vegetable components. However, it's important to eat plain grain at least half the time, since a strongly seasoned grain dish, consumed day after day, can bring too much salt onto your plate. One of the ways to get variety in your diet without its getting too salty is to combine whole grains. Start to play and you will see the myriad of combinations available to you.

Rice goes with just about anything, so barley, millet, rye, spelt, oats, quinoa, amaranth, bulghur, or wheat berries with rice all taste great. Rice with rye is my personal favorite. Some people like 80 percent rice with 20 percent other, but I prefer a 60/40 mix. Millet and quinoa go great together, and don't rule out a three-way, using rice, barley, and wheat. Yowza.

Whole grains are incredibly versatile, but some guidelines do apply. Many grains need to be soaked before cooking or they just won't soften up. Other grains are better, and more digestible, when soaked, but don't have to be. Still others taste best when they are dry-roasted in a skillet or saucepan for a few minutes before boiling (for dry-roasting directions, see recipes on p. 88 and p. 90). Many grains can be pressure-cooked, although usually in combination with rice. You will find recipes in some macro books for baking grains in the winter. Tables 2 and 3 list instructions for boiling and pressure-cooking the most common grains.

a pinch of salt

We need to get something clear right up front. A "pinch of salt" means something very particular in this book. Whereas your mother may have thrown a small handful of salt into a dish as a pinch, our pinch is the following: with *dry* fingers, pinch some salt. What is caught between the pads of your thumb and finger—not what might stick to them—is the pinch. Unless specified otherwise, we use one pinch of salt per cup of grain. This is not a huge amount of salt, as you will see, but salt is such a powerful food that it's important to learn to respect it. The more finesse you have around salt, the better cook you will be.

TABLE 2: BOILING INSTRUCTIONS FOR WHOLE GRAINS			
GRAIN	PREP NEEDED	WATER-TO-GRAIN RATIO	BOIL TIME
Brown rice	Soaking preferred	2:1	50 minutes
Barley	Soaking preferred	2:1	45 minutes
Buckwheat	Roasting preferred	2:1	20 minutes
Millet	Roasting preferred	3:1	30 minutes
Oats	Soaking needed	2 to 4:1	50 minutes
Quinoa	Roasting preferred	2:1	25 minutes
Amaranth	None	3:1	30 minutes
Whole wheat	Soaking needed	2:1	50–60 minutes
Spelt	Soaking needed	2:1	50–60 minutes
Rye	Soaking needed	2:1	50–60 minutes
Hato Mugi	Soaking preferred	2:1	45 minutes
Teff	None	4:1	30 minutes

LET ME BE YOUR CHEWRU

Now that you have learned about grains and are beginning to think of how to prepare them, let's stop for a minute and consider how to eat them. According to macrobiotic teachings, you should chew each mouthful of food between fifty and one hundred times.*

I was in a health-food restaurant in New York a while back, and a woman sitting across the room leaned over to her mate, with a sneaky, judgmental look

---

*In the name of holy lineages, I have my own Chewru; his name is Lino Stanchich, and he's a good friend and great macrobiotic counselor who wrote a book called *The Power Eating Program: You Are How You Eat*. I highly recommend it.

TABLE 3: PRESSURE-COOKING INSTRUCTIONS FOR WHOLE GRAINS

GRAIN	PREP NEEDED	WATER-TO-GRAIN RATIO	PRESSURE-COOKING TIME
Brown rice	Soaking preferred	1½:1	50 minutes
Barley	Soaking preferred	1½–2:1	40 minutes
Buckwheat	Roasting preferred	1½–2:1	Only when prepared with rice
Millet	Roasting preferred	2:1	20–25 minutes
Oats	Soaking needed	1½ to 4:1	30–40 minutes
Quinoa	Roasting preferred	1½:1	Only when prepared with rice
Amaranth	None	2:1	Only when prepared with rice
Whole wheat	Soaking needed	1½:1	50 minutes
Spelt	Soaking needed	1½:1	50 minutes
Rye	Soaking needed	1½:1	50 minutes
Hato Mugi	Soaking preferred	1½:1	40 minutes
Teff	None	2–4:1	n/a

on her face, and whispered, "*Psss ss sssss* macrobiotic *pspspppsss* chewing so much," as she glared at me as I was spacing out, with my fork down, remasticating my cud.

I knew exactly where she was coming from: somewhere along the line, she had read a book on macrobiotics that told her to chew every mouthful of food one hundred times. "Jeez, Louise," she thought. "Enough, already! Rice, I can handle. Even organic vegetables make sense. Yin and yang are quite a stretch, but chewing a hundred times? You've got to be kidding!" This is where macrobiotic people really look like a bunch of freakin' weirdos.

And she's right. Chewing is weird. Chewing is disgusting. Chewing does not lend itself to scintillating conversation. Chewing is a pain in the butt. But you won't get all the insanely wonderful benefits of eating good food without chewing at least some of the time.

Here's why: the digestion of complex carbohydrates (grains and vegetables) begins in the mouth. We secrete an enzyme called ptyalin, which needs to be mixed well with the food. This mixing happens only through chewing. And if the food is not well broken down in the mouth, other digestive enzymes along your gastrointestinal tract cannot work as well. The whole system gets messed up, and you don't absorb the goodness from the food.

Plus, when you chew, you're actually crushing the food into tiny pieces. As you break down the molecular structure of the food, all the energy, vitamins, and minerals of the food become available to your body. Uncrushed, they get sent down the digestive tract in their pseudo-whole form, their insides never used by the body. This uncrushed food causes fartiness and is just dead weight that the body either stores or flushes out, either way requiring unnecessary energy for no real benefits.

But wait. We're not finished yet. One of the greatest benefits of chewing well is that your saliva, which is alkaline, begins to alkalize the food. And one of the whole concepts behind macrobiotic practice is keeping the blood in a slightly alkaline condition. To make that happen, chewing is necessary.

When you chew a mouthful of rice one hundred times, it becomes sweet because it is breaking down into glucose in your mouth. What you're left with is an exceptionally sweet liquid with little bits of fiber floating in it. The liquid is perfect fuel for your body. It will be absorbed magically and happily by your small intestine, elevating your blood sugar in a smooth and balanced way, allowing your pancreas a rest, and it will register a type of satisfaction in your brain that is totally amazing.

I used to be a compulsive overeater. I ate and ate and never felt satisfied. After a huge meal, I still had cravings for more food. The reason this happened was that, although I was chucking a lot of food into my mouth, I was absorbing almost none of it as useable energy for the present moment. It got stored or dumped. My blood sugar (the determiner of a feeling of energy and satisfaction) only got raised when I ate white sugar, and that caused my pancreas to secrete unnatural amounts of insulin to balance it out. So as soon as I had a little high, my body—in its attempt to keep me healthy and balanced—pulled me down again. Hard. At which point, I craved more sugar. Satisfaction eluded me. But then I started to chew. . . .

Being truly nourished is not about the amounts, or what we eat, or even the quality. It is *how* we eat that determines whether the food gets in and does its thing. Try it. You'll be amazed.

It doesn't work just because chewing takes so long you get bored with eating (although that happens). It's not just that you chew right past those magic twenty minutes needed for the brain to register fullness (although that happens, too). It works because, for the first time in your life, you're actually eating. The food is finally going in as the fuel that it is.

And you don't have to chew every mouthful. I only chew about a third of what I eat because I like to have conversations with other human beings during mealtimes. I eat on the run sometimes, and I just get sick of being so conscious around food. Also, if I'm really, really hungry, it's difficult to relax into chewing until my stomach has stopped growling. But a third of my food is enough to give me that feeling of satisfaction, delivers good energy, and keeps me nourished.

However, whenever I want to shed a few pounds, I chew every mouthful of food one hundred times. In a few days, not only is the weight gone, I feel light and springy because I haven't been tossing rocks down my body. I also chew extremely well before acting in a play or making a speech. I have gotten rid of constipation and indigestion by chewing. Finally, chewing is my secret weapon for a hot date. You see, when all the food I eat enters me as liquid, the energy of my whole being is smooth and liquidy—I feel sexy, confident, and totally alive. Try it—you'll thank me. Now let's get cooking!

Perfect Brown Rice

Okay, so maybe that's a little arrogant. But this is a standard, and very trustworthy, way of making good brown rice. And to be quite honest, just as potters spend a lifetime perfecting the art of "centering" a slab of clay on the wheel, macrobiotic cooks are always using their rice as a litmus test for their own attentiveness, sensi-

tivity, and general condition. In other words, it's never perfect; it's just this day's mirror of you and the universe. Whoa. Deep.

- 2 cups short- or medium-grain brown rice, soaked in spring water overnight if possible
- 4 cups spring water
- 2 pinches sea salt

Whether soaking or not, rice always needs to be washed and checked for hulls, bugs, and rocks. So to begin, examine the rice for foreign matter and discard it. Then, in the cooking pot (preferable a heavy one), cover the rice with water. Swirl the rice and water around with your hand a few times and then pour off water through a strainer, so as not to lose any rice. Repeat this rinsing one more time. Don't worry if the water seems cloudy. The murkiness is the result of natural starch, and we don't want to rinse it all away.

If soaking the rice, measure out the amount of water needed for cooking and pour it on top of the rice. Let sit 3–12 hours and cook in soaking water.

If not soaking, simply add the cooking water and bring to a boil, uncovered, over medium heat. When it is boiling, add salt, reduce heat to low, place on flame deflector, cover with heavy lid, and simmer 50 minutes. Turn off heat and let rice sit 5 minutes to unstick from bottom of pot. Fluff with wooden spoon and serve.

SERVES 6

Pressure-Cooked Brown Rice with Chestnuts

I find this to be one of the most satisfying, yet simple, macrobiotic dishes I know. The chestnuts give a lovely texture and sweetness to the rice, which is a grain that loves to be pressure-cooked.

- 1 cup dried chestnuts, soaked in 2 cups spring water overnight if possible
- 3 cups brown rice, soaked in spring water overnight if possible
- 4½ cups spring water (including chestnut-soaking water)
- ½ teaspoon sea salt

Before cooking, remove as much brown or red skin from the chestnuts as possible. Place rice, chestnuts, and their soaking waters (making up 4½ cups of liquid total) in the pressure cooker. Bring to a boil over medium-high heat. Add salt, close the pot, and bring to full pressure.

Place flame deflector under pressure cooker, reduce heat to low, and let cook 50 minutes (pressure cooker should hiss very quietly). Remove from heat and let pressure come down naturally. Open and serve.

SERVES 6–8

Variation

If you do not have time to soak the chestnuts, wash and roast them over a medium flame. Be sure to continually stir them, to avoid burning. They are ready when they are golden brown, softened, and smell sweet.

Mediterranean Barley Salad

Harriet McNear was a wonderful woman and a great asset to the macrobiotic community. She ran a cooking school out of her home in Florida, where she hosted chefs from around the world and showed how their recipes could be made with healthier ingredients. It was on a trip to visit her that I tasted this amazing dish. Harriet was opinionated, funny, and never afraid to live fully. She passed away a few years ago, but I definitely feel her spirit in the kitchen.

Dressing
- 2 tablespoons fresh lemon juice
- 1 tablespoon Dijon mustard
- Pinch sea salt
- 2 tablespoons sherry vinegar *or* 1 tablespoon apple-cider vinegar plus 1 tablespoon umeboshi vinegar
- 1 tablespoon minced shallot
- ¼ cup olive oil

Salad
- 5 cups spring water
- 2 cups pearl or hulled barley
- ½ teaspoon sea salt
- 2 bay leaves
- 2 tablespoons chopped fresh oregano *or* 2 teaspoons dried and crumbled
- ⅓ cup pitted and chopped Kalamata olives
- ⅓ cup drained capers
- ½ cup toasted pine nuts
- ¼ cup finely chopped green onions

To make dressing, combine all ingredients in a mixing bowl or dressing bottle and set aside.

To prepare salad, bring water to a boil. Add barley with salt and bay leaves. Simmer for 1 hour or until all water is absorbed. Cool and add dressing and oregano. Chill about 2 hours or until ready to serve. Before serving, add olives, capers, pine nuts, and green onions. Serve.

SERVES 6–8

Rice, Avocado, and Corn Salad

Avocados are not a regular food on the macrobiotic diet for people living where they don't grow. However, for people in good health, the occasional avocado or guacamole in the summer is fine, and this recipe was just too delicious to leave out of the book.

Dressing
- 1 tablespoon lemon juice
- 1 tablespoon olive oil
- 1 tablespoon brown rice vinegar
- 1 tablespoon shoyu

Salad
- ½ cup almonds
- Kernels from 2 ears corn
- 2 avocados
- 3 cups cooked brown rice
- 2 dill pickles, diced
- ½ small red onion, finely chopped

To make the dressing, mix the lemon juice, olive oil, vinegar, and shoyu in a bowl or dressing bottle and set aside.

To roast the almonds, you can either put them on a baking sheet for 8–12 minutes in a 350°F oven or pan-roast them in a heavy skillet over medium-low heat for about the same amount of time. If you pan-roast, make sure to keep the almonds moving continually to avoid burning.

They're ready when they're easy to break open but are still cream colored in the center. Don't wait for the centers to get tan colored—that's a sign they're a little burnt. After roasting, let almonds cool and then chop roughly. *P.S.* You can also buy almonds roasted (and unsalted) at the store.

Slice avocados in half, remove pits, spoon out flesh, and mash thoroughly into rice. Bring a pot of water to a boil and blanche the corn kernels for 1 minute. Remove with slotted spoon and let cool. Add pickles, nuts, onion, and corn to the rice mixture. Add dressing and mix well. Let sit for about 30 minutes to let the flavors blend.

SERVES 6

Good Morning Oat Porridge

Oats are so strong, they make horses run, fast. Whenever possible, it is preferable to eat whole oats rather than cracked or rolled oats because their vital energy remains intact. Oats always make me feel nourished and comforted.

- 1 cup whole oats
- 4 cups spring water
- Pinch sea salt

Before bed, bring oats and water to a boil. Let simmer, uncovered for 5 minutes. Turn off heat, cover, and go to bed. In the morning, bring the mixture back to boil. Add the pinch of salt and more water if necessary. Reduce heat and let simmer over flame deflector for 45 minutes. Serve.

SERVES 4

Quinoa Salad

Howard and I found this recipe in MacroChef *magazine, a macrobiotic journal put out for many years by Christina and Robert Pirello. You can now get her recipes at christinacooks.com or in her cookbooks. This salad was a big hit every time we made it.*

- ½ medium red onion, cut fine into half-moons
- 4 radishes, cut fine into half-moons
- 2 tablespoons umeboshi vinegar
- 1 tablespoon brown rice vinegar
- 1½ cups quinoa
- 3 cups spring water
- ¼ teaspoon sea salt
- ⅔ cup hazelnuts
- ¼ cup chopped parsley *or* chopped mint
- ½ cup raisins, washed and drained

Mix the onion and radishes with both vinegars. Place a plate and weight on top, and press for 1 hour to pickle. Wash quinoa thoroughly with water to remove the bitter saponin on the outside of the grain. Roast in a dry heavy-bottom fry pan until dry, stirring constantly until grain begins to turn golden and puff up a little.

Bring water and salt to a boil in a saucepan, stir in quinoa, cover, and bring back to a boil. Turn the flame down low and simmer until all the water is absorbed (about 20–25 minutes). Remove from heat, fluff with a fork, and turn into a mixing bowl to cool.

Wash and roast hazelnuts at 325°F until nuts are golden and skins crack and loosen. Rub the nuts in a dry dishcloth to remove any loose skins. Chop roughly. Mix hazelnuts, quinoa, onions, radishes, herbs, and raisins together, including pickling liquid. Serve.

SERVES 4

Variation

Yummy if not yummier. Substitute pearled (polished) barley for quinoa (it also needs 2 parts water to 1 part grain, simmered for 30 minutes). Replace hazelnuts with toasted pecans, use dried apricots that have been soaked and chopped instead of raisins, and add fresh chopped dill at the end to replace the parsley or mint. You still use the red onion and radish pressed with the vinegars.

Millet Mashed "Potatoes" with Mushroom Gravy

It's such a bummer that potatoes are a deadly nightshade (see discussion of nightshades on p. 141). Although I still get french fries every once in a while, I no longer cook potatoes in my home. This recipe, creamy and satisfying, mimics great mashes from childhood.

- 1 cup millet, washed
- 3 cups water
- 2 cups cauliflower, in small florets or medium-sized chunks
- Pinch sea salt

Gravy
- Toasted sesame oil
- 1 medium onion, diced
- Pinch sea salt
- 12 white button mushrooms *or* 8 fresh shiitake *or* 6 dried shiitake
- About 2 cups spring water
- ¼ cup shoyu
- 2 tablespoons mirin

- 1 drop brown rice vinegar
- 2 tablespoons kuzu, diluted in ½ cup cold water
- Scallions or parsley for garnish

Place the washed millet in a heavy 2-quart pot. Over medium heat, stir the millet continually until it dries and then becomes aromatic and ever-so-slightly golden in color. This can take 5–8 minutes. Add water and cauliflower. Bring to a boil. Add salt. Cover and simmer over a flame deflector for 30 minutes. Remove from heat. Put millet through a hand food mill or blend in a food processor or in the pot with a handheld food processor. Blend to desired creamy consistency.

To make gravy, heat toasted sesame oil over medium heat in a skillet. Add onion, salt, and sauté until translucent. Add mushrooms and sauté until soft and moist. Add water and bring to a boil. Season with shoyu, mirin, and brown rice vinegar. Simmer 5 minutes. Adjust seasonings to your taste, and simmer 5 more minutes.

Add diluted kuzu to simmering mixture and stir constantly as kuzu thickens and comes to a boil. After the kuzu has boiled, the gravy is ready. Spoon over millet mash on individual plates and serve. Garnish with scallions or parsley.

SERVES 4

Variation
Add a small beet in addition to the cauliflower. When blending, this will turn these "potatoes" a fantastic pink that the kids will love.

Fried Basmati Rice

- 1 red pepper
- 1–2 tablespoons toasted sesame oil
- 1 onion, diced
- 1 pinch salt

- 1 carrot, diced or cut into matchsticks
- Dash umeboshi vinegar
- 2 cups cooked basmati rice
- 1–2 teaspoons shoyu
- 3 tablespoons spring water
- 10 snow peas, sliced into medium pieces
- Kernels from 1 ear corn *or* ½ cup frozen corn
- 1 scallion *or* a small amount of watercress, chopped

Roast the red pepper over a medium flame, turning often to blacken it all over. Place it in a paper bag for 10 minutes to let it sweat. Remove from bag and peel off skin. Cut into slices and then dice.

Heat oil over medium heat in skillet. Add onion, a pinch of salt, and sauté until translucent. Add carrot and sauté 2 minutes. Add red pepper and a dash of umeboshi vinegar, to preserve its red color. Mix in rice and season with shoyu. Sprinkle water and place snow peas and corn on top of rice. Cover and let cook 5 minutes. Mix with scallion or watercress. Serve.

SERVES 2–4

Variation

There are endless possibilities for additions here: mushrooms, broccoli, pine nuts, leeks, summer squash, red cabbage . . . you name it. Or add Indian spices to make it more aromatic.

Amaranth and Apricots

This delicious breakfast porridge has a strong flavor and texture that might take a little getting used to, but once you know it, you will love it.

- 8 apricots
- 1 cup organic apple juice
- 1 cup amaranth

- 2 cups water
- 2 tablespoons organic raisins
- 1 pinch salt

Soak apricots and raisins in apple juice for at least 1 hour. Slice apricots into medium-sized strips. Mix fruit and apple juice with amaranth and water in a pot and bring to a boil. Add salt. Cover and reduce heat. Add flame deflector. Let simmer 30 minutes. The consistency will be sticky and weird, but I think you'll like it.

SERVES 3–4

Kasha and Cabbage

- 2 cups spring water
- 1 pinch sea salt
- 1 cup roasted buckwheat
- 2 tablespoons sesame oil
- 1 cup diced onion
- 2 cups red cabbage, in large dices
- 1 tablespoon umeboshi vinegar
- 1 teaspoon caraway seeds
- ½ cup sauerkraut juice
- ½ cup chopped parsley

Bring water and salt to a boil. Add buckwheat. Let it return to a boil, then cover, reduce heat, and simmer 15–20 minutes over a flame deflector. Turn off heat. Let sit 15 minutes to let grains unstick from bottom of pot. Remove lid and fluff. Set buckwheat aside to cool.

Heat oil in skillet over a medium flame. Sauté the onion and cabbage, adding umeboshi vinegar to retain the purple color of the cabbage. Add caraway seeds and sauté until the vegetables are quite limp, about 5 minutes. Stir in the cooled buckwheat and mix thoroughly. Add the sauerkraut juice, stir, cover, and reduce heat. Simmer for about 1 minute to absorb the juice. Toss in parsley and serve.

SERVES 4

MOVING ON TO PHASE TWO

Phase Two is for people who need to wade in the shallows a little before diving into the deep end. In this phase, we concern ourselves not so much with balancing yin and yang forces in the kitchen but with learning about extreme yinners and yangers—the foods that eventually need to be minimized for optimal jiving with the Infinite Universe. We'll be looking at why they're considered extreme, the pros and cons of eating them, and the ways in which you can replace them and stay happy.

Hopefully, you've been eating whole grains for a little while now. Whole grains, given the opportunity to calm your nervous system, balance your blood sugar, and clear your mind, have begun to chart a new course for your eating and your life. If you've just been reading up until now, remember to incorporate whole grains as a principal food in your daily eating while you explore Phase Two.

Be bold. Embrace change. Eat whatever else you want, but be willing to learn about food and cook some new things. Try the following recipes. Get familiar with your health-food store. Eating whole foods is one of the most powerful and exciting choices you will ever make in your life. Trust that your body and soul want to feel good and are willing to do whatever it takes. Don't hold them back. Life's too short to deprive yourself of freedom. Go for it. Now.

CHAPTER SIX

phase two: cupboard conversion

Each food we eat has both yin and yang qualities, but—since nothing in the universe is neutral—every food is either more yin or more yang, and all foods have their place relative to other foods on the continuum of yin to yang. Chart 1 describes these relative relationships.

There are a few things you should know about Chart 1. First, it is not exact. A graphic depiction can only show so much. For instance, how you cook something changes its yinness and yangness, so there's no fixed yinness or yangness.

Second, just because one item is near one end of the chart does not mean that it is necessarily balanced by the opposite item on the other end. For example, macrobiotic cooking uses salt, which is—as you can see—very yang. But that doesn't mean that drugs balance salt or that salt balances drugs. Their relationship in the picture does not represent their relationship in the material world.

Third, there are different types of yinness and yangness. For instance, there is yinness due to wetness and yinness due to upwardness. There is yangness from density, yangness due to sodium content, and yangness that produces dryness (to name a few.) Although it is generally depicted in this fashion, a linear representation of foods between yin and yang is not dynamic enough to tell the whole story. Let this be only an initial guide as you discover the rest of the story through your experience.

Finally, it is from between the lines that we choose the majority of our daily foods. The exception is salt, which is so yang that it is at the end of the chart but is used in small amounts. Some of the other foods and substances that fall outside the lines are used by healthy people, in moderation, on occasion, but none of them is considered supportive for restoring health; they exist for sensory pleasure and play. Too much food taken from the extremes will erode your health, so go easy.

CHART 1: THE YIN AND YANG OF FOOD

MORE YIN

Drugs

Alcohol

Sugar

Spices

Liquid, creamy, sweet dairy

Tropical fruit and nightshade vegetables

- -

Fruit juice

Fruit

Sea vegetables

Vegetables (upward)

Vegetables (round)

Vegetables (downward)

Beans

Grains

White-meat fish

- -

All other animal food and

salty dairy

Eggs

Salt

MORE YANG

the extremes

What a great name for a band! Drew Barrymore would probably date the drummer. In this section, we're going to look at foods that most of us have been taught to eat. Each has its own particular impact, not necessarily good or bad, just extreme. Macrobiotic cooking uses foods that are less energetically extreme and foods that represent the expansion and contraction models in nature. So—although life definitely requires that we do extreme things sometimes—these foods are not meant for regular consumption.

Macrobiotics is about saying "yes" to life, to freedom, and to a host of new foods. So after each section, I have included delicious recipes that use ingredients that aren't extreme to replace the foods that are. The last thing I want is for you to see macrobiotics as deprivation and negation, but it's difficult to discuss the extremes, most of which we all grew up on, without being a little negative. So just as it's easier to forget an old boyfriend when a new guy comes along, let yourself walk toward the new foods instead of getting all hung up on the old.

red meat (beef, pork, etc.)

I hate poo-poohing meat. Not because I'm a meat lover, but because there has already been such vitriolic, hysterical, arrogant meat-bashing in the last hundred years that I hate to get on the bandwagon. I do not think eating animal food is inherently bad. I don't think eating anything is inherently bad, as long as I remain aware of the effects and what I'm learning from them. I certainly think when any food is eaten—animal or vegetable—the best mindset is to remain deeply grateful for the source, for that food is becoming me and I am becoming it. It is determining my next move.

Having said all that, meat is an incredibly intense food. And we eat a lot of it. It is only in the last century or so that we have had the wealth, the transportation, and the refrigeration required to get so much meat into so many individuals. In the West we tend to eat a lot of muscle meat, as opposed to the organs. In Asia, this seems weird, because they see the internal organs as being full of life force, whereas the muscles are just the errand boys of the nervous system.

It may be no accident that we have developed a culture in the last few hundred years that has an increasing obsession with the flexing of muscle; we go to the gym in numbers that grow every day. Even the term *working out* implies an underlying energy—twitchy, punchy muscle energy—that needs to be discharged. We love to watch movies of people punching people. The image of the ideal man, strong and protective, is one packed with layer after layer of hard-earned muscle. We don't project men as needing to be flexible and wise. We have even developed a new neurosis, wiggling its way into the psyches of the gym addict, called "muscle dysmorphia," whereby he (or she) no longer recognizes any reasonable limit to the expansion and development of new muscle. Sort of a reverse anorexia. Yikes. The following are the energetic qualities of red meat—both hurtful and helpful—that you should know in order to choose what's right for you.

MEAT IS VERY YANG

Because it is the concentrated (yang), blood-infused (yang), heavy (yang) product of chewing, digestion, and the magical alchemy of the animal's body, meat is extremely yang. Animals are very hot, dense, concentrated, and complex beings, compared to the cool, peaceful plants most of them eat. (Even *they* don't eat meat!) This yangness produces strong energy that needs to be discharged, usually physically. Because animal protein has very little water in it (compared to plants) and produces lots of internal heat, meat-eaters get thirsty a lot, and the recommendation to chug six to eight glasses of water is designed for a meat-eating nation (this is also because animal protein builds up uric acid in the human body, and fluids are needed to create urine in order to discharge it). If you choose to eat red meat, you will crave some sort of extreme yin like potatoes, tomatoes, sugar, or alcohol in order to balance its yangness. This makes for a very long and teetering seesaw.

MEAT IS ACID FORMING

Although red meat is yang, it also produces strong acids in the body. Red meat creates a type of acidity that—because meat is heavy and dense—gravitates to the lower regions of the body, affecting the intestines and reproductive organs. Any acidity within the body calls for mineral stores to buffer it; therefore, meat can deplete your mineral stores, contributing to such nasty health conditions as osteoporosis.

WE ARE NOT DESIGNED TO EAT A LOT OF MEAT

When we look at the small intestine of the human body, we see that it is about four times longer than that of the average carnivorous dog. Because our intestines are so long, dense animal protein tends to become acidic and putrefy during the extensive trek toward defecation. This long gut is designed to absorb mostly vegetable-quality foods. Our teeth tell a story too: of thirty-two adult teeth, only four are designed for doglike flesh-ripping (appropriately called our canines). This seems like a message from the universe that our intake of animal food need not be more than one-eighth our total intake of food.

MOST MEAT IS HIGH IN SATURATED FAT

Saturated fat is the grandfather of sludge. If you don't know what it is, look at your roast beef drippings after they have cooled. The waxy, yellowish hard stuff is saturated fat. In macrobiotics and the medical community, it is believed that saturated fat (and the meat it's attached to) contributes to hardening of the arteries. Stroke, heart attack, hypertension, and cholesterol are all produced by excess yang and are related to grandpappy sludge.

ANIMAL FOOD SUPPORTS
AGGRESSIVE BEHAVIOR

Notice I wrote "supports," not "creates." There are some people who eat lots of red meat who have never thrown a punch in their lives. But how many boxers do you know of who are vegetarian? Because eating animal is eating muscle, it makes for muscle-y discharge. One way to do that is to go to the gym. A lot. Another way is to deck somebody. Or invade a country.

EATING MEAT SUPPORTS SELF-CENTEREDNESS

Now this is a touchy matter. Let's put it this way: yangness is about contraction, and without some contraction, nothing would get done. But extreme contraction creates a spiral that can become closed and egocentric. From meat-eating, we get the cult of the individual. The self becomes a type of god, and the whole is rarely perceived as an organic entity to which the individual belongs. Instead, there is a sort of cowboy mentality and a society of "Leave me alone and I'll leave you alone." Now don't get me wrong—I'm all for the self. But the self is the antagonistic and complementary opposite to the whole, and one cannot exist without the other. It is the essential paradox of humanity that we exist as individuals, within groups. Both our individuality and our groupness need to be honored and nourished at the same time. Whole grains feed the self, while leaving the eater sensitive to the whole, while the saturated fat of meat tends to dull the individual to the vibes of others and the vibes of the whole.

Finally, red meat is so yang that it leaves little space within the individual for patient self-reflection. Meat's twitchy, hot energy supports impulsive, sometimes compulsive, behavior. We need to slow down and be still in order to tune in to the vibes of the universe, which is re-creating and directing us every day, but meat will not allow for that. It's no accident that most yogis and meditators lean toward vegetarianism.

ANIMAL FOOD CAN MAKE SEX COMPULSIVE AND REDUCE OVERALL SENSITIVITY

I'll go into this later in the book, but suffice it to say that saturated fat and the extreme yang tightening of red meat can make the individual energy system less available for the amazing vibrational exchange that is sex. Also, the buildup of testosterone that occurs from eating so much muscle can create a real urgency around sexual energy and even lead to premature ejaculation.

EATING MEAT DOESN'T FEED YOUR BRAIN

Your brain needs blood sugar—that's its fuel for thinking and envisioning your dream in life. Meat is mostly minerals, protein, and fat, with absolutely no carbohydrates to make blood sugar. Yes, low-carb diets will cause your fat to convert to glucose, which feeds the brain, but after that's all gone, you're running on meat as a primary food.

So meat gets you to work, takes you to the gym, and rents that dirty video, but it doesn't feed your ability to receive refined vibration and think holistically. In fact, meat keeps us so yang in an animal sort of way that we become strongly tethered to the material world, less apt to enjoy the human gift of conscious connectedness with the Infinite Universe.

MOST MEAT IS PUMPED FULL OF HORMONES

Most dairy cattle are slaughtered after they have been pumped full of (1) hormones to make them get bigger or to lactate up to *twenty times* more than normal, and (2) antibiotics to cure any number of funky conditions, including the really painful cases of mastitis that they get from hyperlactation. After this miserable slavery, the cow is used for her beef, which is now *full* of sludge. And don't get me started on the sludge created by Bessie's own nervous system, in the form of stress hormones pumped into her bloodstream, thanks to her lousy life. You're not just eating a cow—you're eating a *dysfunctional* cow.

Our "innocent until proven guilty" credo in this country makes some sense in a court of law determining the consequences of human behavior, but it doesn't really stand up in the Infinite Universe. There is no "guilt" or "innocence" in the order of the universe. There is just cause and effect. Yin and yang. The bigger the cause, the bigger the effect. Every action has an impact. We can spend many years, millions of dollars, and a ridiculous amount of energy trying to "prove" that pumping animals full of garbage is not dangerous, but we are simply fashioning cataracts for our intuition. Is it rational to think that we can push one of nature's organisms (a cow) so beyond its natural energy template and not have that extreme continue through the food chain? Can you drop a stone into a pond and create no ripple? I believe that the sludge in commercial meat affects us in a very negative way.

However, macrobiotics is not vegetarian. It is not strictly anything: it is about you and your relationship to the Infinite Universe. You are free to choose. So what are the advantages of eating animal food?

ANIMAL FOOD PROVIDES STRONG, WARM, AND LONG-LASTING ENERGY

Meat is good for physical strength and for maintaining an aggressive "edge" in the world. Meat eaters tend to get things done. Considering that macrobiotics is about understanding the energy of food and the freedom to use it wisely, it makes sense to use some kind of animal food if your lifestyle and your goals demand it. You may need some strong energy to do your job, play rough-and-tumble with the kids, or run that marathon, but you probably don't need red meat three times a day, every day, to give you that. A little fish'll do.

GUIDELINES FOR MEAT EATERS

Given all that I've said above, it seems that organic, lean meat—in moderate amounts—makes the most sense for those who choose to eat it. However, know that its yangness will seek yinness, and be prepared to balance it with good-quality sweets, lots of fresh salad, or some alcohol. If you feel you need red meat, understand that it delivers a very strong punch and that even one serving a week will yangize your energy. Men may feel they need a little more, because they are governed by yang force. If you decide to go "whole hog" macro for a while, fish is the only animal food considered mild enough to be balanced by other macrobiotic foods. If you are considering using the macrobiotic diet to address a health issue, red meat will be thrown out of the picture because it is considered simply too yang.

MEET THE NEW MEAT

Tempeh

Much of what attracts people to meat is its density and richness. Meat is heavy and satisfying. Although tofu is usually seen as the meat substitute of most healthful eaters, let's face it: tofu just doesn't cut it as a red-meat substitute. However, it has a cousin that does: tempeh (pronounced *tem-pay*). Tempeh is indigenous to Indonesia and is a fermented food (although versions sold in stores have been pasteurized). Made of split soybeans fermented combined with a special starter, tempeh is rich and dense. It is sold in eight-ounce packages like thin bricks. It is also a very good source of protein. When it's homemade, and therefore unpasteurized, tempeh is an excellent source of vitamin B_{12}. It can be made with just soybeans, or with other ingredients like grains, vegetables, or sea vegetables. For the following recipes, you might want to start with the plain.

Seitan

Seitan sounds evil, but it tastes great. Seitan (think "suntan" but with a "say") comes from the gluten of kneaded wheat flour, which looks like a heavy, spongy blob and sounds totally disgusting. However, after the blob is cooked in yummy broth, it firms up and has a meaty texture and flavor. It is packaged and sold in health-food stores—although hard-core macros make their own—and is perfect for stews or other meaty dishes.

Tempeh Burritos

- 1 8-ounce package tempeh
- 2 cups water
- ½ cup shoyu
- 3 tablespoons mirin
- 1 dash brown rice vinegar
- Toasted sesame oil or light sesame oil

- 1 small onion, diced
- ½ teaspoon salt
- ½ teaspoon chili powder
- ½ teaspoon garlic powder
- Whole-wheat tortillas
- Soy cheese, grated
- Tofu Sour Cream (see recipe on p. 122)

Cut tempeh into four chunks and bring to a boil in the water, shoyu, mirin, and brown rice vinegar. Let simmer 20 minutes. Set aside.

Meanwhile, over medium heat, coat a skillet generously with oil. Sauté onion with salt, until onion is translucent.

Crumble up cooked tempeh into bits like ground beef and sauté with the onion. The tempeh should be well seasoned, but keep the cooking liquid just in case you would like to add a little more later. Stir in chili powder and garlic powder. Allow whole concoction to cook for about 5 minutes. The tempeh should absorb lots of the oil and may even get a little crispy.

Warm a tortilla in another skillet. Add "beef" and some grated soy cheese. Wrap tortilla around filling and let it warm on the skillet so that the soy cheese melts. Serve with Tofu Sour Cream and/or guacamole.

Variation

Also great as a filling in tacos! Feel free to Mexicanize this dish to your personal taste. For a really authentic burrito, add refried beans.

MAKES 4 BURRITOS OR TACOS

Tempeh Reuben with Russian Dressing

Russian Dressing
- 2 tablespoons fruit-sweetened ketchup
- 2 tablespoons organic relish
- ½ cup Tofu Mayonnaise (see p. 123)

Tempeh
- 1 8-ounce package tempeh (feel free to use different types, like three-grain tempeh or quinoa sesame)
- ½ cup water
- 2 tablespoons shoyu
- 2 tablespoons toasted sesame oil
- 4–8 slices whole-grain sourdough bread
- 1 tablespoon unsweetened sauerkraut or any unsweetened pickle

Mix dressing ingredients together by hand and set aside.

Chop block of tempeh in half. Simmer tempeh in water and shoyu until liquid is absorbed—about 15–20 minutes. Flip tempeh at least once so that each side gets seasoned. Pan-fry tempeh in sesame oil until crispy. Steam bread (in a steamer for 1 minute (or grill it in a little olive oil until crispy). Slice tempeh in half and place tempeh, sauerkraut, and dressing on two pieces of bread. Place top slices on sandwiches. Slice and serve. Great additions are lettuce, sprouts, or raw red onion.

SERVES 2 *(although if you slice*
the tempeh in half widthwise,
you can make 4 slimmer sandwiches)

Seitan Stew

This is a great stew for cold winter days. Warms you right up!

- 1–2 cups seitan, cut into big bite-sized chunks
- 3 cloves garlic, cut into small pieces
- 1 medium onion, cut into thick wedges
- 2 carrots, cut into large diagonal chunks
- 1 stalk burdock, sliced on a thin diagonal
- 1 cup brussels sprouts, cut in half
- 1 stalk celery, cut on a thin diagonal
- Spring water
- ¼ cup shoyu
- Kuzu, diluted in ⅓ cup cold water

Place the seitan and garlic, onions, carrots, burdock, brussels sprouts, and celery in a 6-quart pot. Add spring water to just cover, then add shoyu. Bring to a boil. Reduce flame to low and simmer until vegetables are done, about 20 minutes. Add diluted kuzu, stirring constantly until it thickens the stew. Simmer 5 more minutes. If the stew is too thin, add a little more thickener. If too thick, add more cold water for desired consistency.

SERVES 4–6

on tofu hot dogs, veggie burgers, etc. . . .

When at a barbecue, I go for the tofu hot dog or the veggie burger in a flash. At this point, my digestion can handle them much better than it could real meat.

However, I have to continually remember what my friend Lisa tells her classes: "If you can't pronounce it, you probably have no business eating it." These products can be full of unpronounceables, often in the form of added vitamins and minerals. But the earth doesn't produce nutrients in capsule form or as free-floating entities to be jammed into "health-food" products. Nature produces whole foods, and the vitamins and minerals therein are balanced and absorbable when eaten in their original package. When we break a natural organism into bits and pieces, extracting this and that, we create imbalance in the organism. When we then feed ourselves these extractions for added nutritional oomph, we create imbalances in ourselves. If you are eating a varied, balanced macrobiotic diet, you should be getting all the nutrients you need.

I don't keep prepackaged health products in the house, and I don't make them regular choices. In terms of energy, it is arguable that an organic hamburger could be a better-quality choice than a processed food containing lots of chemicals, even when it is labeled "veggie" or "health food." Of course, it is up to you to eat whatever works for you, but don't become hypnotized by everything the "health" industry says.

chicken and eggs

In our culture, chickens look like the good guy next to red meat, the bad guy. Lighter in color, lower in fat, chicken's gotten a pretty decent rap. In macrobiotics, all dualities are reduced to yin and yang, and chicken is neither good nor bad, but it is certainly yang. And everything I said about red meat above goes for chicken. With one exception: chicken is *more* yang than red meat. Think of it this way: imagine a cow next to a chicken. Which one is bigger, slower, and more expanded? Which one is smaller and more contracted, and moves more quickly? The chicken wins every time. Chicken energy is very intense, twitchy, and can be a little neurotic. Chickens are known for a precise pecking order and aggressive behavior toward one another, especially when cooped up for long periods of time, which most of them are. Chicken energy, so tight and compact, tends to gravitate toward the center of the body and can tighten especially the middle organs like the pancreas, contributing to blood sugar imbalances.

These days, because chicken is considered the "good" meat, chicken eaters eat lots and lots of it with impunity. Ever notice people with chickenish noses? Or birdlike haircuts?

Eggs are—energetically—whole chickens in a shell. Which makes them *more* yang than chicken. A three-egg omelette has the vibrational template of three entire chickens in it. They are considered so powerful that, in Asian cooking, when eggs are used, they are spread thinly throughout a dish—like in pad thai or in a soup—as opposed to being the principal food. An egg is a chicken ovum, and some macrobiotic people believe that egg energy is attracted to and gathers at the ovaries in female egg-lovers.

Although I have an egg every blue moon (or come across one in Asian restaurant cooking), eggs are generally not in daily macrobiotic cooking because they are considered so difficult to balance effectively.

If you choose to continue to eat eggs and chicken, or feed them to your family, definitely get organic, free-range chicken and organic eggs. They are more expensive, but the absence of hormones, chemicalized feed, and ridiculous fowl aggression is well worth it.

THE NEW CHICK IN TOWN

Here comes the tofu! This soft, cold block of tasteless soybean curd has been the unwitting poster child for the health-food industry for the last thirty years. Poor tofu. Such expectations! So maligned. So misunderstood.

So let's clarify: because tofu has very little taste, it immediately picks up the flavors of the foods around it and blends in like an elegant, well-mannered guest. Tofu is also misunderstood because some vegetarian people tend to make it their only, and daily, source of protein. This is a mistake, because quantity affects quality. You see, tofu is cold (yin), soft (yin), and made of soybeans (yin), and therefore it is quite a yin food. It is excellent for keeping cool in the summer and even as a topical remedy for treating burns. Tofu is also rich in phytoestrogens and good for menopausal women. However, eat too much tofu and an overall cooling can take place, which is not good for anyone, but especially not good for the sex drive of a man (which depends on heat a little more than a woman's). But don't get freaked out: Tofu in moderation, which means a couple of servings a week, is generally fine for everyone and won't put the kibosh on your love life.

Tofu is also not a whole food, because the soybeans have been crudely processed, so it doesn't deliver the more whole protein of the bean alone. Use tofu, but don't forget to eat other beans and bean products as well.

Christina's Chickenless Chicken Salad

Christina Pirello is an amazing teacher, chef, and redhead. I highly recommend all her cookbooks, and this recipe is adapted from her Cooking the Whole Foods Way. *You* must *try this.*

- 1 pound extra-firm tofu
- Shoyu
- Spring water
- 3 celery stalks, diced
- 1 small red onion, diced
- 1 red bell pepper, roasted over an open flame, peeled, seeded, and diced
- ½ teaspoon each basil, sage, rosemary, and oregano
- 2 teaspoons paprika
- 1–1½ cups Tofu Mayonnaise (see p. 123 or store-bought)

Preheat oven to 400°F. Lightly oil a baking sheet. Cut tofu into ¼-inch-thick slices. Place slices in a shallow dish and cover with a mixture that is 1 part shoyu to 4 parts water. Allow tofu to marinate 10 minutes. Place tofu slices on oiled baking sheet and bake 30–35 minutes or until deep golden brown and crispy on the outside. Remove tofu slices from oven and allow to cool until you can handle them.

Shred the tofu slices with a sharp knife, creating irregular, angular pieces similar to shredded chicken. Mix with vegetables, spices, and tofu mayo until ingredients are coated. Chill thoroughly before serving.

SERVES 4

Tofu "Egg" Salad

- 1 pound firm or extra-firm tofu
- ½ cup Tofu Mayonnaise (see p. 123 or store bought)
- ¼ cup tahini
- ¼ cup minced red onion
- ¼ cup minced dill pickles
- 1 tablespoon umeboshi vinegar
- 1 tablespoon organic Dijon mustard
- 1 teaspoon shoyu
- ½ teaspoon mirin
- ½ teaspoon turmeric
- ⅛ teaspoon black pepper (optional)

Boil the tofu for 5 minutes to make it more digestible. Set aside and let cool. Mix together all other ingredients and crumble tofu into it. Mix thoroughly and serve.

SERVES 4

Tofu Quiche

This original recipe is by Lisa Silverman, who runs the 5 Seasons Whole Foods Cooking School here in Portland, Maine. Whenever she makes it, I find some way to invite myself over for lunch.

Crust

- 1 tablespoon olive oil
- 1 clove garlic, minced
- 1 small onion, diced
- Pinch sea salt
- 1 tablespoon fresh rosemary
- 1 cup millet, washed
- 3 cups spring water

Filling

- 1½ pounds tofu
- 3 tablespoons tahini
- 2 tablespoons umeboshi vinegar
- 2 tablespoons olive oil
- 1 onion
- 2 cloves garlic, minced
- 2 tablespoons fresh rosemary
- Pinch sea salt
- ¼ pound destemmed and sliced fresh shiitake mushrooms
- 4 tablespoons shoyu

Preheat oven to 350°F. Heat olive oil in 2-quart saucepan. Sauté garlic and onions, adding a pinch of salt. Add rosemary and sauté 3–5 minutes. Add millet and sauté 1 more minute. Add water, bring to a boil, and then simmer 30 minutes over low flame with flame deflector.

Meanwhile, mix tofu, tahini, umeboshi vinegar, and 1 tablespoon of the olive oil in food processor until smooth. Remove from food processor and place in large bowl. In a skillet, heat the other tablespoon of olive oil over medium heat and add onion, garlic, rosemary, and a pinch of salt. Sauté until onion is translucent. Add shiitake mushrooms and sauté until they soften. Season with 3 tablespoons of the shoyu. Add this vegetable sauté to the tofu mixture.

When millet is done, press it into an 8-by-8-inch baking dish moistened with water to prevent sticking. Spread tofu/vegetable filling over millet crust. Sprinkle the remaining tablespoon of shoyu on top of filling to help it brown. Bake for 30 minutes. Let cool for 30 minutes before serving.

SERVES 4–6

fish

I wish we knew more about fish. Because today's bodies of water are so compromised by industrial sludge, God only knows what we're getting in our fish. We've gotten hip to mercury levels, but that's just one potential hazard in the mix. The good thing about fish is that because it is so low on the food chain, it's lower in fat and is a much less complicated organism than a chicken, a pig, or a cow and, therefore, does not contain sludge in the same concentration as other meats do. Of the animal foods, fish is easiest to digest. Whenever possible, buy fish that is caught wild and fresh; farm-raised fish almost always contains antibiotics, and fish loses lots of its energy and freshness when frozen.

Fish, like all the other animal foods, supports active, physical energy. Macrobiotic cooking tends to use white-meat fish because it is lower in fat and less yang. If you are in good health, don't be afraid to shake things up with some salmon or tuna every once in a while. It helps to get things done and keep up with the rest of the twenty-first-century world. But fish should always be balanced with green, upward-growing vegetables. And it's not unusual to serve a lemon wedge, dessert, and/or a beer at fish meals as well. Raw daikon (always served with sashimi in Japanese restaurants) helps to break down the heavy fats found in some fish.

Fried Fish Wraps with Asian Coleslaw and Rice

When Lisa Silverman first made this dish for me, I gave her what I considered the highest compliment: "This tastes just like fast food!" For some reason, most chefs don't appreciate that. The combination of the fried fish and the "mayo" in the coleslaw creates a wonderful, rich, and delicious taste. Enjoy.

Asian Coleslaw

- ¾ cup Tofu Mayonnaise (see p. 123 or store-bought)
- 2 teaspoons dark sesame oil
- 1 tablespoon umeboshi vinegar
- 1 tablespoon brown rice syrup
- 1 cup shredded red cabbage
- 1 cup shredded green cabbage
- ½ cup shredded carrots
- ½ bunch cilantro, chopped

Fish

- 1 pound white fish (such as haddock or flounder)
- 2 tablespoons shoyu
- 1 tablespoon mirin or sake
- 1 tablespoon brown rice vinegar or grated fresh ginger
- 1–2 tablespoons sesame oil
- 1 cup cornmeal
- 1 lemon wedge (optional)
- 4 whole-wheat tortillas
- 2 cups long-grain basmati rice, cooked

To make the Asian coleslaw, combine tofu mayo, sesame oil, umeboshi vinegar, and brown rice syrup in a large bowl. Add slaw mix and cilantro and blend well. Set aside for 1 hour.

Place the fish in a dish and cover with the shoyu, mirin, and vinegar. Marinate for at least 1 hour. Remove the fish, cut into three-inch pieces, and roll in a little cornmeal. Heat a skillet on a medium flame and add the oil. When the oil is hot, add the fish and fry for 2–3 minutes on each side or until the fish is tender and golden brown in color. Drain on a paper towel. Squeeze a little lemon juice on the fish if desired.

Heat tortillas on a skillet. Arrange rice, fish, and coleslaw on tortillas and wrap. Serve.

SERVES 4

dairy food

I know I just said, all egalitarian and open-minded, that no food is either bad or good. That was all very groovy of me, and for the most part I believe that, with one exception: dairy is, pretty much, bad for you. That feels good. Remember what we thought about cigarettes sixty years ago—that they were relatively harmless? And what we know now? Well, hopefully, we will see the same turnaround about dairy in the next sixty years. Generally, people don't like to hear that. They don't like to equate their nightly ice cream with evil, evil nicotine. But not only is that an apt analogy, but eating the dairy food of another species is quite possibly *more* harmful than smoking. In fact, it can be argued that dairy consumption, which tends to accumulate in the lungs (among other places), is a bigger contributor to lung cancer than cigarettes. The smoke needs the mucky, snotty, wet deposits that dairy leaves in the lungs in order to make nice, deadly tumors.

WE AREN'T COWS

Think about it. Dairy food is the baby food a cow produces for her calf, just as human women produce milk for their babies. Human children, left to their own devices, naturally wean themselves when they make the transition to healthy, solid food. Even baby cows don't eat their mother's milk past infancy. Why are baby cows smarter than we are? How do they build such big bones, such muscle mass, and produce such vast amounts of milk, without continuing to drink milk themselves? Where do they get the calcium to do that? Why are we nursing on Bessie the cow as thirty-, forty-, and fifty-year-old adults? What the hell are we doing?

DAIRY STRESSES OUT THE BODY

Now don't get all freaked out about the grated Parmesan cheese on the salad you ordered at the restaurant last night. It's not like one ounce of dairy is toxic or that it is going to kill you. It's not like plutonium or SARS. It's just that your body will have to find a creative way to handle any dairy you ingest, because, as the baby food of another species, it has no business being inside of you. Your body doesn't have a natural relationship to it, and therefore it either gets coughed up as phlegm; pushed out as oil and zits; packed onto your breasts, hips, and belly; or, worst-case scenario, curdles itself into a nice little stagnating cyst.

Lots of people's bodies have no lactase (the enzyme specifically designed to break down lactose) anymore, so they can't really digest dairy comfortably. When I say lots of people, I mean, oh, millions of people in Africa, Asia, and the Caribbean. These cultures have also managed to grow strong people, with strong bones, many living to very ripe old ages without our miracle food, dairy. You see, our guts were meant to let go of lactase after we are weaned, because there is no real reason to keep it. We lose it the way we lose our baby teeth. Isn't nature economical? One theory is that the cultures that have continued to produce lactase do so because our collective histories required at some point, whether it was because of drought or duress, that we lean on the milk of our friend the cow. Because milk was necessary for pure survival at certain points, our bodies, perfectly adaptable and fitted for our survival, decided to digest it again. Considering our circumstances today, that is no longer necessary for the majority. In fact, chronic colds, allergies, ovarian cysts, menstrual cramps, infertility, kidney stones, obesity, and breast cancer could represent our version of lactose intolerance.

Finally, sadly and tragically, the new wave of obese children, along with their precociously pubescent friends, may be suffering from the freaky amounts of growth and sex hormones to which we subject our dairy slaves. (Ooops! I mean cows!)

MILK INHIBITS YOUR RELATIONSHIP TO THE INFINITE UNIVERSE

Milk is cloudy—for your body, brain, and spirit. It is dense and created for physical nourishment, not spiritual nourishment. Milk is the food that nature designed to bond a baby with its mother, for security and safety. It actually contains hormones that do just that. So if you're eighteen months old, that's great. Dairy foods are so sludgy that they literally produce a cloudiness, like a cataract, that inhibits your direct relationship to the Infinite Universe. Your skin, chakras, and organs accrue a layer of sludge that inhibits the vibes coming in from heaven and earth. The sludge of dairy even inhibits your taste buds from picking up the subtleties of healthy foods. So reserve your final judgment of macrobiotic cooking until you've been off of dairy for a few months. Whole grain has a direct relationship with heaven and earth, the sun and the air, with no physical mother relationship in between, so the connection forged with whole grains is direct. The hotline to the universe.

DAIRY FOOD SLOWS YOU DOWN

Cows aren't speedy animals, and they're not known for their precision. You'll find, after eating whole grains and eschewing dairy for a little while, that your whole being sort of clears up and speeds up. Energy will pass through you unimpeded, at what feels like lightning speed.

DAIRY CAN BE HARD TO GIVE UP

Don't get down on yourself if, while reading this, you're thinking, "Holy cow, I don't want to give up *dairy!* I love dairy!" Don't worry. Every dairy lover feels the same way because you are literally, physically, and hormonally bonded to dairy as you are bonded to your mother. One of the biggest reasons we should get off it is the reason it's so hard. However, you will find, as you grow spiritually by eating whole grains, that a strength develops beyond what dairy could deliver, and then you will discover that it becomes much easier to let it go.

DAIRY IS BOTH VERY YIN AND VERY YANG

Dairy food that is more liquid and lighter, like milk, is more yin. Milk or cream combined with sugar and fat and frozen (any guesses?) is *extremely* yin. Milk that is combined with salt, as in heavy sauces or cheese, is more yang. Yin dairy has a tendency to accumulate in the upper regions of the body, like the breast tissue, lungs, and lymph. Yang dairy is heavier and collects more in the lower body and reproductive organs.

DAIRY DOESN'T GIVE YOU THE
CALCIUM YOU THINK IT DOES

Technically, the dairy pushers are not lying to you. Yes, cow's milk has lots of calcium in it—more than human milk. But what they're not telling you is that cow's milk also comes with a large amount of phosphorus, which binds with the calcium in our digestive tracts and makes most of the calcium unabsorbable. The ratio of calcium to phosphorus in human milk is such that the phosphorus actually helps the calcium to be absorbed. Again, nature has designed human milk perfectly for human bodies. So even though cow's milk looks like the winner in the laboratory, it's actually the loser in the body.

The osteoporosis crisis in our culture is not so much about a lack of calcium; it is more about ingesting substances that create acid in the blood, which requires your stored calcium in order to buffer it. They include coffee, alcohol, soda pop, vinegar, citrus, sugar, nightshade vegetables, dairy food, meat, and tobacco. Familiar with any of them? When these substances are refrained from, calcium and other minerals are allowed to stay at the party in your body. Then sources of absorbable calcium, like leafy greens, sea vegetables, nuts, seeds, beans, and whole grains can do a most excellent job keeping your bones strong.

DAIRY IS BIG BUSINESS

We were all brought up to believe that dairy is the perfect food because there is a big ol' National Dairy Council that has made it its job to create that belief. Sugar is big business, too. So are tobacco, oil, and meat. Get a nation of 300 million people to become dependent on your product for their entire lives because they fear for their teeth and bones, and you've just made a lot of money. Cows don't tend to question what they're told, but you can.

IS DAIRY GOOD FOR ANYTHING?

Good question. Dairy wins a gold medal in the category it was designed for: it is excellent and perfect for babies, setting a kid up immunologically and emotionally *much* better than formula ever could or will be able to. Its ability to deepen the bond between mother and child is one of nature's most precious miracles. But calves should get cow's milk and babies should get human milk. If you have the choice, breast-feed your babies. Let your milk do the job that no other food can do.

Because it is fermented, cheese is easier to digest than plain milk and imparts (if unpasteurized) good-quality bacteria to the gut. But the benefits of fermentation are available in lots of other foods as well, like miso and pickles.

Because dairy is so comforting, it may be an appropriate choice for things like birthday cakes or foods you bring to funerals. And you may want to slather frosting all over your body once in your life to turn on your beloved. Go for it!

SOY CHEESE, MILK, ICE CREAM, AND MARGARINE

These products sound ideal, don't they? And some of them are mighty tasty. But just as with tofu hot dogs and veggie burgers, these products need to be processed (and chemicalized) in such a way that they are about a million miles away from a soybean by the end of it all. Plus, they're pretty sludgy. Most soy cheeses contain casein, which is an animal product that makes the cheese very difficult to digest completely. Soy milk can also be hard to digest, leaving lots of people bloated and gassy. And if those things don't convince you, maybe this will: after I stopped drinking soy milk and eating soy cheese, ice cream, etc., a whole layer of fat that had never budged before simply disappeared!

Soybeans are yin to begin with, and after adding all the other stuff and refining them to the hilt, these products become *extremely* yin (although soy cheese has lots of salt, so it's more yang). This yinness makes them acid forming and, over time, weakening. Don't get into the habit of eating cereal with soy milk every morning thinking that you're desludging your body. It is simply health food's version of sludge. Yes, sometimes I'll put soy cheese in a burrito. Yes, I will make a soy milk smoothie every once in a while, but they are only very occasional foods. Ditto rice milk, oat milk, and almond milk bought at the store.

But don't despair. We have lots of good stuff to satisfy your dairy needs. In macrobiotic cooking, we use foods that can be prepared to deliver that creamy, yummy, satisfying texture of dairy, without the sludge. Tofu, mochi, amazake, tahini, and various other things, in different combinations, will be your new comfort foods. You won't miss dairy after a while, I promise.

Rice Dream Chocolate Sundae

Okay. I just dissed rice milk a little, too. However, this recipe is for people (like me) who just have *to have something from our pasts once in a while. I loved ice cream so much as a kid that the people at my local Baskin-Robbins, thinking I was older than I was, offered me a job at eleven years old! Needless to say, when I found Rice Dream, I thought I had died and gone to heaven.*

Rice Dream is an ice-cream substitute that is made from rice. It has no dairy and no white sugar. This recipe, because it includes Rice Dream, vegan chocolate syrup, Hip Whip, and is cold, is very yin. Have some to counter those yang feelings when you're feeling very wound up and need to relax, or after a meal with an-

imal food. Eating this regularly will cool you down and expand you too much, creating weakness. I probably have Rice Dream about once a month. All cold foods dampen natural kidney energy, and in Oriental medicine the kidneys are related to courage and will. They are also related to sexual vitality, so go easy.

- 2 scoops vanilla or strawberry frozen Rice Dream
- 1 large dollop Hip Whip (a health-food nondairy topping sweetened with brown rice syrup)
- 2 tablespoons fruit or malt-sweetened chocolate syrup (available in most big health-food stores)
- 1–2 tablespoons chopped walnuts or almonds (may be lightly roasted)

Scoop the Rice Dream into a bowl and add the Hip Whip on top. Over low heat, warm up the chocolate sauce and drizzle on top. Garnish with chopped nuts. I haven't figured out the maraschino cherry yet, but maybe you will.

SERVES 1

Tofu "Cheese"

This is great for parties, served on crackers, or just as a snack to remind you of the texture of cheese.

- 1 pound firm or extra-firm tofu
- 1 cup miso (the darker the miso, the darker and stronger the "cheese")

Wrap the tofu in a paper towel, place a plate and weight on top of it, and press the excess liquid out of the tofu for 20 minutes. Remove the paper towel and wrap the tofu in one layer of cheesecloth. Apply miso to completely envelop the tofu, about ¼- to ½-inch thick. Place in a bowl and cover with cheesecloth. Let sit for 2, 3, or 4 days, depending on the strength of flavor desired. When done, remove the cheesecloth and rinse the tofu in cold water. Slice and serve.

SERVES 6–8

smoothies

Some people live out of their blenders these days. If you are one of them, consider these recipes to acquaint yourself with some new ingredients.

Lisa's Mango Laasi

- 1 mango, pitted and chopped
- 1 cup soy milk*
- ½ teaspoon vanilla
- ½ teaspoon ground cardamom
- 1 tablespoon maple syrup

Blend all ingredients together. Yum!

SERVES 1

*Be sure to use soy milk that is either unsweetened or sweetened with rice syrup or barley malt. The fewer unpronounceables, the better.

Your New Chocolate Milk Shake

- 1 cup soy milk or plain amasake
- 1 tablespoon almond butter

- 1 tablespoon dairy-free, fruit-sweetened chocolate syrup or topping
- 1 ripe banana
- ¼ teaspoon vanilla
- ¼ teaspoon umeboshi vinegar
- 1 drop mint extract (optional)

Whiz ingredients in blender and enjoy.

SERVES 1

Fruit Smoothie

- 1 cup oat milk
- ½ cup pineapple juice or coconut milk
- ½ cup fresh or frozen peaches
- ½ cup fresh or frozen blueberries
- ¼ teaspoon vanilla
- ¼ teaspoon umeboshi vinegar

You know what to do.

SERVES 1

Tofu Sour Cream

- 1 pound soft tofu
- 6 tablespoons sunflower oil
- 2 tablespoons fresh lemon juice
- 2 scallions, white part only

- 1½–2 tablespoons umeboshi vinegar
- ¼ teaspoon sea salt

Blend all the ingredients in a blender or food processor and serve with burritos, tacos, or any other dish that deserves it.

Tofu Mayonnaise

This recipe makes the best quality "mayo," so it's good to have some on hand. It will last about a week in the fridge.*

- 8 ounces soft tofu
- 4 teaspoons umeboshi vinegar
- ¼ teaspoon sea salt
- Juice of 1 lemon
- 1 tablespoon organic Dijon mustard
- 1 tablespoon brown rice vinegar

Place the tofu in boiling water and let simmer 5 minutes. Allow it to cool a little. Place all the ingredients in a food processor and blend until very smooth. Chill and use.

MAKES 1 CUP

---

*If you occasionally choose to use store-bought vegan mayonnaise made with tofu or grape-seed oil, check the label carefully for evaporated cane juice or various unpronounceables. I use the kind with brown rice syrup and the most natural ingredients.

Lasagna

I'm not Italian, but I think I've made a pretty good vegan lasagna here. It takes some time, so I only make it on special occasions, but it lasts a couple of days and it's totally worth the effort.

Chunky Tofu Ricotta
- ½ pound extra firm tofu, crumbled
- 1:1 dilution spring water and umeboshi vinegar (for marinade)

Smooth, Firm Tofu Ricotta
- 1 pound tofu
- 1 small handful fresh basil
- Approx. 1–2 tablespoons extra virgin olive oil
- Approx. 1–2 tablespoons tahini
- Umeboshi vinegar to taste
- Shoyu to taste

Carrot/Beet Sauce
- 4 large carrots, cut into chunks
- 2 medium onions, cut into wedges
- 1 winter squash, cut into chunks
- 1 small beet
- Spring water to cover
- ½ teaspoon sea salt
- 2 tablespoons olive oil
- 3 cloves garlic, minced
- 1 pinch sea salt
- 1 large onion, diced
- 1½ cups sliced mushrooms
- 1 stalk celery, sliced
- Italian spices to taste

- Shoyu to taste
- Umeboshi vinegar to taste

Noodles
- 1 pound white or whole-wheat lasagna noodles

Additional Items
- Sautéed portobello mushrooms
- Sautéed or blanched summer squash or zucchini
- Blanched broccoli
- Seitan

Mochi Cheese
- 8 ounces grated or thinly sliced mochi
- Spring water to cover
- Shoyu to taste
- Umeboshi vinegar to taste

CHUNKY TOFU RICOTTA: crumble tofu and let sit in marinade for 1 hour.

SMOOTH TOFU RICOTTA: put first four ingredients in blender. Blend until smooth. Then add seasonings until it tastes good to you. Set aside.

CARROT/BEET SAUCE: in a pressure cooker, place carrots, onions, squash, and beet. Add water to almost cover. Add salt. Close and bring to pressure. At full pressure, reduce heat to low and let cook for 20 minutes. Remove from heat. Let pressure come down. Open pressure cooker and transfer vegetables and some of the cooking water to a blender or food processor. Blend until smooth, adding liquid if necessary, re-creating the texture of tomato sauce. When all the vegetables are blended, set the sauce aside.

In a skillet, heat olive oil over medium heat. Add garlic and a pinch of salt. Sauté for about 10 seconds and then add onion, sautéing until the onion becomes translucent. Add mushrooms and sauté until they soften, about 3 minutes. Add celery and sauté 1 minute.

Now pour pureed vegetables into skillet with sautéed vegetables. Add Italian spices like dried basil, oregano, or marjoram, to your taste. Season with shoyu and umeboshi vinegar to create the tomato-y taste that works for you. Let the whole concoction come to a boil, then simmer over low heat, covered, for about 15 minutes.

Boil the lasagna noodles according to the directions on the box. While noodles boil, prepare any additional lasagna ingredients you desire, like sautéed portobello mushrooms, zucchini, broccoli, summer squash, or seitan.

MOCHI CHEESE: right before layering lasagna, place mochi in a saucepan with water to almost cover. Heat, stirring regularly, until mochi melts. Season with shoyu and umeboshi vinegar to get your desired taste, adding more water if necessary to get a creamy, cheesy consistency. Pour into lasagna layers, but reserve some for the top.

In a large lasagna dish, layer the lasagna, beginning with carrot/beet sauce, then noodles. Then do whatever order suits you, but I like smooth ricotta, carrot/beet sauce, vegetable or seitan, mochi cheese, chunky ricotta, noodles. Repeat until ingredients are used up. Bake covered with foil in oven at 350°F for 45 minutes. Then remove foil covering and let bake 15 more minutes. Let the lasagna sit at least 30 minutes before serving. Even better the next day.

SERVES 8

sugar

There are a whole lot of products out there today pretending *not* to be sugar. They include dextrose, maltose, Florida Crystals, and evaporated cane juice. All these items are sugar renamed, like calling a checkout person a "sales associate." Turbinado sugar, although it retains some of its minerals, is still highly refined cane sugar.

I used to be a sugar junkie. And these days, my ex–drug of choice is getting a bad rap. Recently, popular high-protein, low-carb diets have done a great job in educating the public that refined carbohydrates and simple sugars are not really foods at all and, to add insult to injury, contribute to our expanding girths. But sugar is not a baddie simply because it converts to fat, which converts back to glucose, when necessary. In fact, you could argue that—in terms of pure survival—that's quite a neat trick.

Plus, not all carbohydrates are alike; in fact, what we cavalierly refer to as "carbs" these days covers a range of foods that go from downright devilish to totally life-giving, like whole grains. Distinguishing between good-quality and lousy-quality carbohydrates is a key to good health. As human beings, we need complex carbohydrates to function, and especially to think and experience our spirituality.

Using macrobiotic thinking, it is important to look at the yinness and yangness of things, and sugar, in any form, is yin. It expands us, relaxes us, and has an initially upward-rising energy in the body. But it is the degree of yinness and the speed with which the sugar reaches that expansion that matters. In a nutshell, highly refined sugars will create massive expansive energy very quickly and stress the body out in a number of ways while doing it because extreme yin becomes extreme yang. Less-refined sweeteners made from fermented complex carbohydrates, like brown rice syrup, barley malt, and amasake, take a longer time to hit the bloodstream and don't take us on quite the roller-coaster ride. Maple syrup and molasses (used occasionally in macrobiotics) also contain lots of minerals to help metabolize them well. So don't think your sweet tooth is gonna starve. In fact, sweetness, in macrobiotics, is about much more than taste. Sweet foods impart a soothing, relaxing, and restorative energy to the body and soul. Sweets make us happy and sweeten our personalities. If you include grains and some vegetables among foods that break down into glucose, and are therefore "sweet," macrobiotic cooking should be made up of 80 percent sweet foods! I love that!

WHITE SUGAR LEECHES YOU OF MINERALS

Refined sugar is a thief. Period. Where dairy is adding unnecessary gunk to your closets, sugar is sneaking jewel after jewel out of your treasure chest. You see, when your body is faced with sugar to digest, it provides all the missing bits and pieces taken away in the refinement of sugarcane. So you add your personal store of minerals to the mix. So it's not even that sugar is a thief. Sugar is like a bad guest that comes to your home and does a giddy little jig in the living room for about fifteen minutes, creating a great euphoria in the whole family. Suddenly the dance ends, she picks up an ax, and proceeds to smash and slash all the furniture in the house. The family, so sleepy at this point, cannot stop her. Just before she finally leaves, you say "Wait," run to the bedroom, grab your diamond necklace, shove it in her hands, saying "Here, this is for you" and wave her off with a weary, sad smile. You then do your best to pick up the pieces of the trashed living room and move on. The craziest part is that within a day, you can't wait to have that "little sweetie" over again, so you call her up for a repeat performance. This leeching of minerals contributes to anemia, osteoporosis, and anxiety, among other things. With sugar, we lose B vitamins, calcium, phosphorus, iron, and peace of mind.

SUGAR CAUSES MOOD SWINGS AND DEPRESSION

Sugar is so yin that it raises your blood sugar dramatically. Because yin attracts yang, your pancreas spews out yang insulin in order to balance the extreme of the yin sugar. But it has to send out so much insulin that it then has to balance itself with yin anti-insulin in order to restore some semblance of order. This blood-sugar roller coaster is taking place not only in your blood but also in your brain, which is the biggest user of sugar in your body. This physical drama creates the wonderful ups and downs of the sugar blues, which reminds me of the great book *Sugar Blues,* by the late William Dufty—a must-read for any sugar junkie.

SUGAR PRODUCES ACIDIC BLOOD

Our blood should be slightly alkaline, with a Ph of approximately 7.4. When sugar steals the alkaline minerals from your blood, it becomes acidic, and an overall weakening begins to take place wherever your blood goes—which is everywhere. Sugar doesn't just rot your teeth. Sugar rots everything. Viruses, cancer, and all other types of illness love an acid environment like a good hotel.

SUGAR IS EXTREMELY YIN

It creates expansion within your system and inflammation is a product of expansion. Inflamed joints are painful. Inflamed muscles can constrict nerves, causing pain. Inflamed organs are a very serious thing. Any time there is inflammation (and I have heard it argued that all pain is caused by some kind of inflammation) it is caused by extreme yin, usually sugar, alcohol, drugs, tropical fruits, or nightshade vegetables. Sugar is so expansive that it can contribute to chronic spasms, scattered thinking, and is considered a major player in mental illnesses like Schizophrenia. (In his book *You Are All Sanpaku,* George Ohsawa said, "Sugar is without question the number-one murderer in the history of humanity." Yikes. Talk about extreme!)

SUGAR IS ADDICTIVE

A substance is considered addictive if you have identifiable cravings for it and suffer withdrawal if it is taken away. Most people recognize cravings for sugar, because sugar keeps asking for itself. As soon as your blood sugar drops, you want nothing more than the sugar that caused the problem in the first place. This blood-sugar roller coaster may be the underlying factor in every addictive behavior. Depression, compulsive behavior, and scattered thinking may seem like hallmarks of your personality but are probably just a result of the muffin you're eating.

If you have never kicked sugar before, you may not know the withdrawal it puts a human through: depression, lethargy, intense cravings, anger, negativity, night sweats, nightmares, crying. After thirty-odd years, I have learned how to get off sugar relatively gracefully; I know to eat lots of natural sweeteners to satisfy the cravings. I meditate more than normal to keep myself together. I sit through the profound lows and trust that they will pass.

Be extremely gentle with yourself as you let go of sugar. It may not happen all at once, and you may need a buddy to go through it with. You may get off and then get on again. Don't worry. As you eat whole grains and vegetables, chewing them well, your taste for the strong stuff will lessen. When I eat white sugar now, I am amazed at how strong it is. And at the same time, it's sort of boring tasting, like an orchestra playing one note all evening. Now that my body is accustomed to healthier sweets, it prefers them.

Be gentle in weaning your kids as well. Make good-quality and strong sweets for them at home, using maple syrup and malt-sweetened chocolate. Kids are very yang (small, fast, warm) and crave a lot of yin. If they can get good-tasting sweet stuff at home, they won't go roaming for it quite as compulsively at a friend's house.

SUGAR LOVES MEAT, AND MEAT LOVES SUGAR

Think of sugar as the prom queen and meat as the high-school quarterback—they're perfect for each other and practically inseparable. Because animal flesh is made up of only protein and fat (and is extremely yang), missing its friend the carbohydrate, and sugar is make up of only carbohydrate (extremely yin), missing protein, minerals, and fat, they are the Fred and Ginger of the food world. When you eat meat, you crave either sugar or alcohol. When you eat sugar, it would make sense to ground yourself with meat.

I have met many people who eat a meat-and-sugar diet who, with strong constitutions, look fine and feel fine in their daily lives. They are striking a balance, albeit using extreme components. Over time, this extreme dance creates deep issues, but it can certainly move people through the material world if they are strong to begin with.

However, when a vegetarian or vegan eats lots and lots of sugar, the situation becomes out of balance more quickly. Someone who refrains from animal food does not have the yang of meat to balance the yin of sugar, and so the demineralization that sugar creates becomes exaggerated. A diet replete with white flour and white sugar can be more harmful to a vegetarian than a meat eater, and severe malnourishment problems may occur.

SUGAR MESSES WITH YOUR INTUITION

We need strong, mineralized blood (yang) in order to attract the subtle vibrations of the universe. Sugar is so demineralizing that cane-juice junkies can be completely cut off from their true source, the sweetness of the infinite. Without the ability to pick up their intuition, they lose their direction in life and may never tune in with their true dreams and ambitions. It wasn't until I got off sugar that I really saw—with any clarity—who I was and where I was going.

SOME QUESTIONABLE SUGAR ALTERNATIVES

Stevia

Stevia is an herb that is indigenous to Paraguay. It is recognized as a food additive in the United States but not yet approved for use in foods. Stevia is extremely sweet and has no calories, so it sounds like a terrific answer to saccharin and aspartame. And perhaps it is a much better alternative to chemical sweeteners. It is, however, being tropical and refined, very yin. If you are making a slow transition to macrobiotics and the other sweeteners don't appeal to you yet, use stevia sparingly. If you choose to go whole hog, it's considered extreme.

Artificial Sweeteners

Much is suspected or known about the dangers of artificial sweeteners such as aspartame and saccharin. They are chemicals with extreme, including cardiogenic, effects. It's pretty darn difficult to use these substances and stay in tune with natural rhythms. Just do an Internet search on these substances to get scared stiff. I don't use them.

Maltitol, Xylotol, Sorbitol, and Mannitol

These substances are all known as polyols and are produced through the catalytic hydrogenation of high-maltose corn syrup. They are highly refined and therefore extra yin and far from whole. I figure if I can't understand the process and couldn't do it in my own home (I don't have a catalytic hydrogenator—but maybe this Christmas—fingers crossed!), I shouldn't put it in my mouth.

MACROBIOTIC SUGAR ALTERNATIVES

There are a number of ways to get a sweet taste using healthy foods. In macrobiotic cooking, rice syrup and barley malt are the yummy grain-based sweeteners. Amasake is a thick and delicious drink made from fermented sweet rice. Fruit juice, as well as fresh and dried fruits, also delivers a healthy dose of yumminess. Maple syrup is used occasionally as well. Although all these ingredients are on the yin side of things, none of them is as extreme as white sugar, tropical sweeteners, or artificial sweeteners.

Crispy Rice Treats

When I played Lady Macbeth, the dude who played my hubby—whom I taunted and abused until he murdered the king—was an actor named Chris Price. I couldn't help but think, through many a rehearsal, that I was playing opposite "Crisp Rice," the main ingredient in this excellent dessert.

- 1 cup brown rice syrup
- ⅔ cup peanut butter (or try almond, cashew, or even hazelnut butter)
- Healthy dash umeboshi vinegar
- Healthy dash vanilla (optional)
- 3 cups crispy brown rice cereal
- Cinnamon, nutmeg, raisins, roasted almonds, peanuts, or cashews to taste (optional)

Over a medium flame, heat up brown rice syrup, peanut butter, vinegar, and, if desired, vanilla, stirring constantly until the mixture is smooth, thinned out, and bubbling a little. Pour cereal into mixing bowl. Add rice syrup mixture to it and blend well with a wooden spoon. Pour into an oiled pan and flatten with a wet spatula. Let cool. Slice and serve.

SERVES 8

Chocolate Peanut Butter Cups

These suckers taste just as good as Reese's.

- 4 ounces firm organic tofu
- 3 tablespoons organic peanut butter
- ¼ teaspoon sea salt
- ½ teaspoon umeboshi vinegar
- ¼ cup maple syrup
- 3 tablespoons maple sugar[*]
- 1 teaspoon vanilla extract
- 2 tablespoons filtered water
- 1 cup dairy-free, malt-sweetened bittersweet chocolate chips[†]
- 1 teaspoon canola oil
- Mini foil baking cups as molds

Bring a pot of water to boil, add tofu, and let simmer for 5 minutes. Remove tofu from water, and let it cool just enough so that you can handle it with your hands. Wrap block of tofu in clean dish towel or paper towel and place on a plate. Put another plate on top of the tofu and add a short, heavy weight in order to press the excess liquid out of the tofu. Press for 15 minutes. Place tofu, peanut butter, salt, umeboshi vinegar, and maple

---

[*]If the filling seems too sweet to you, reduce the maple sugar content.

[†]Chocolate, too, is generally considered an extreme because it is a combination of dairy, sugar, and the tropical substance cocoa. This chocolate doesn't contain the first two, but it's still cocoa and still very yin. Chocolate is not used by people looking to recover their health and only on occasion by those in good health.

syrup in a blender. Blend until smooth. Add maple sugar and vanilla extract. Blend for about 2 minutes, scraping sides when necessary. Refrigerate in a closed container for 1 hour.

In a double boiler, place chocolate chips and oil over boiling water. Stir until the chocolate melts. Turn off heat. With a pastry brush, coat each baking cup along the bottom and up the sides. (If you can't find mini-cups, paint only halfway up a full-sized cup.) Put in freezer until chocolate hardens. Repaint each cup to thicken the chocolate coating. Freeze again. The chocolate hardens quite quickly. When the filling has chilled for 1 hour, spoon some into each cup. If you like, you can then paint over the filling with another layer of chocolate, or leave it topless. When ready to eat, just peel the baking cup carefully away from the chocolate and enjoy. Store in freezer.

MAKES 1 DOZEN PEANUT BUTTER CUPS

white-flour products

White flour is to a grain as heroin is to a poppy. So refined (and usually chemically treated), this very yin white powder basically breaks down into refined sugar in the body and, therefore, does just what sugar does. So see the "Sugar" section to get a handle on white flour. However, white flour does have a couple of its own interesting characteristics.

WHITE FLOUR MAKES FOR SLUDGY INTESTINES

Because it comes with no fiber, your intestines have a hard time working white flour through them: white flour gets gunky and stuck in the tiny little hairlike villi of the intestinal wall. This not only messes you up for digesting flour properly but also inhibits the absorption of all other foods.

WHITE FLOUR MAKES FOR SLUDGY THINKING

In Oriental medicine, the intestines and the brain are energetically linked; what happens downstairs is mirrored upstairs. Just remember the last time you were constipated; blocked intestines lead to an irritable, blocked mind. Or when you fast; empty intestines make for clearheadedness. Well, sludgy intestines make for sludgy, cloudy thinking. White flour is excellent for . . . papier-mâché.

I'm not suggesting that you eschew all white flour for the rest of your life. As you eat more mineral-rich foods like grains, leafy greens, and sea vegetables, on a regular basis, your mineral bank account fills up and you can have that white pasta at your friend's wedding and it's no big deal. But to eat this stuff every day can be very weakening and lead to mood swings, fatigue, and depression.

BAKED FLOUR MAKES YOU CRANKY AND SORE

I know that sounds weird. And I'm talking here about *baked* flour products in particular, as opposed to other flour products like noodles. Unlike a noodle, which is rehydrated in the cooking process, bread that is baked (and other yummy baked "goods") produces dryness. Even whole-wheat baked bread is dry. This quality can leech fluids from you and contribute to an overall tightness that results in neck, shoulder, and upper-back discomfort. Your liver, which is particularly sensitive to baked flour products, can become irritated, and when your liver is irritated, you are irritable and cranky. Check in with your next irrational, angry moment and ask yourself if you've eaten bread in the previous hour. If you suffer from chronic neck and back issues or general lack of flexibility, stop eating all baked flour products (including muffins, corn chips, pretzels, cookies, cake, crackers, pizza, pie—sorry) and the symptoms should lessen considerably.

whole-grain flour

In macrobiotic cooking, when flour is used it is almost always the whole-grain variety. Because whole-grain flour products still contain some minerals and fiber, as well as the starch of the grain, they are more easily assimilated and don't steal minerals from your blood or bones. Keep in mind, however, that whole-grain products are not whole foods; because the grain has been cracked in order to make flour, it has been oxidized, losing much of its energy. So flour products, in general, are never a replacement for the incredible energy of grains, but life without a noodle every once in a while is not worth living! Whole-wheat products include:

- *Bulghur wheat:* This is wheat that has been precooked and cracked, so its energy is no longer whole. But for summer days and lighter meals, it is ideal.
- *Whole-wheat noodles:* Principally udon (whole wheat) and soba (a combination of wheat and buckwheat) are used. Feel free to experiment with corn, quinoa, spelt, and brown-rice noodles.
- *Whole-wheat couscous:* Thank Allah for couscous. So quickly cooked, these tiny balls of pasta can keep your life fast and convenient when necessary.
- *Whole-grain breads:* The bread used most in macrobiotic cooking is whole-wheat, unyeasted sourdough, because commercial yeasts can produce weakness and expansion of the intestines, resulting in a myriad of problems. Look for whole-wheat pita bread that has been unyeasted. Yeast-free tortillas may be a little harder to find, but see what's out there.
- *Sprouted-grain bread:* Usually available in the freezer section of the health-food store, this bread is not actually made of flour but the sprouted grain itself, contains no yeast, and tastes awesome. Good for a quick snack.
- *Mochi:* Technically not a flour, mochi is made of sweet brown rice steamed and then pounded (therefore no longer a whole grain) into a glutenous, yummy "cake" that you then recook by pan-frying, baking, or making it into a waffle. It can also be baked into little "croutons" or grated and melted like cheese on vegetable dishes. Don't let the word *sweet* fool you; sweet brown rice is not sweet like candy—it's just richer and higher in fat and protein than regular brown rice. In Japan, it is given to new mothers to help them lactate. I find that mochi, chewed

well, imparts amazing strength and energy. If included on the Standard Macrobiotic Diet, mochi is fine to eat once or twice a week.

Elegant Orange Couscous

This is an incredible recipe I happened on to as a private chef. It is perfect for warm, summer weather or just as a totally glam accompaniment to fish. The orange juice and the fruit in the couscous make this dish light and yin, balancing the yang energy of the fish.

- 1 cup whole-wheat couscous
- ½ cup spring water
- 1 cup fresh orange juice
- ¼ cup light olive oil
- 4½ teaspoons umeboshi vinegar
- ¼ teaspoon sea salt
- 6 dried apricots, thinly sliced (about ¼ cup)
- 2 tablespoons dried currants
- 2 teaspoons grated fresh ginger
- ¼ medium-sized red onion, finely diced (about ½ cup)
- 3 tablespoons toasted pine nuts

Measure couscous and put it in a medium-sized bowl. In a pot, combine water, orange juice, oil, 4 teaspoons of the vinegar, and salt. Bring it all to a boil and add the dried fruit and ginger. Let simmer for about 1 minute. After a quick stir, pour this liquid mixture over the dry couscous. Stir just to eliminate any pockets of dry couscous. Cover the concoction with a plate or plastic wrap to hold in the heat. The couscous will cook by itself in about 20 minutes.

In a smaller pot, bring about a cup of water to a boil and drop in the diced red onion. Let it boil for 20 seconds. Take the onion out with a slotted spoon or mesh strainer and put aside.

Add ½ teaspoon (the balance) of the umbeboshi vinegar to the onion and mix to bring out its red color. When the couscous is cooked, fluff it with a fork, and then add the onion and pine nuts. Serve.

MAKES 4 LARGE SERVINGS

Tabbouleh

- 1½ cups spring water
- ¼–½ teaspoon salt
- Peppermint tea bag (optional)
- 1 cup bulghur wheat
- ¼ cup olive oil
- ¼–⅓ cup lemon juice
- 2 cloves garlic, minced
- 1 tablespoon chopped fresh mint
- 1 small tomato, diced (optional)
- 1 cup cucumber, diced
- ¼ red onion, sliced finely into half-moons
- ¼ cup kalamata olives, halved
- ¼ cup chopped parsley
- Tofu "Cheese" (see p. 122)

Bring water, salt, and, if desired, the tea bag to a rolling boil. Boil 1 minute and remove tea bag if used. Add bulghur, cover, place on a flame deflector, and reduce heat to low. Let simmer about 15 minutes or until all water is absorbed. Take out of pot and put in bowl to cool. Mix oil, lemon juice, garlic, and mint into a dressing. When bulghur is cool, toss in vegetables, olives, parsley, and dressing to taste. When you have a satisfying taste and texture, chop tofu cheese into bite-sized cubes and carefully fold it in. Serve immediately or chill first. Great with pita bread and hummus.

SERVES 4–6

fruit

In terms of yin and yang, fruit is very yin: expansive, watery, and acid forming. The Standard Macrobiotic Diet includes much less fruit than most others, because it is impossible to eat lots of fruit and keep your blood slightly alkaline. If you want really strong and consistent vitality, fruits are foods that need to be respected as the amazing natural "treats" they are and to be used in moderation. Instead of three servings of fruit every day, I might have one serving every second or third day and maybe throw some apple or raisins into a salad.

One of the basic principles of macrobiotics is seasonal, local eating. Because I live in Maine, I generally stick to fruits that grow in my area: apples, pears, berries, etc. I also eat very little fresh fruit in the winter; instead, I go for cooked fruit, or dried fruit (more yang, as all food should be in winter). So when choosing your natural treats, consider where you live and the time of year. Whenever possible, buy organic, since fruit—being so watery—picks up more pesticides and other chemical sludge than other foods.

Because it takes so much fruit to make a cup of juice, juice is considered very yin. I love a warm cup of apple juice to mellow me out when I'm wound up, and this next recipe uses juice, but again, it is used for specific purposes and in moderation; chugging fruit juice all day like water is very weakening and depletes mineral stores.

Strawberry Kanten with Creamy Topping

Gelled with a sea vegetable called agar agar, kantens are the macrobiotic answer to Jell-O. The word kanten *means "frozen heaven" in Japanese, and although they are not frozen, kantens are certainly heavenly. You will be amazed at how delicious this dessert is, while pleasingly simple. You can do a thousand variations on the basic kanten theme, using different fruits, juices, garnishes, and toppings. In my fifteen years of eating macrobiotic food, I have never tired of kantens; they are delicious, relaxing, soothing, and good for regularity. This pudding is also great without the creamy topping.*

Kanten
- 4 cups organic apple juice
- ¼ cup agar agar flakes
- ¼ cup rice syrup
- Pinch sea salt
- ¼ cup kuzu root starch
- 1 cup fresh or frozen organic strawberries, chopped

Creamy Tofu Topping
- 1 pound firm tofu
- 1 cup rice syrup *or* ⅔ cup maple syrup
- 1 teaspoon umeboshi vinegar
- ½ teaspoon vanilla

Garnish
- ½ cup finely sliced roasted almonds

Bring 3½ cups of the apple juice, agar agar, rice syrup, and salt to a boil. Reduce heat to low and simmer 10 minutes, stirring occasionally until all the agar flakes are dissolved. Dilute the kuzu in the remaining ½ cup of apple juice (this juice must be room temperature or cold in order to dilute the kuzu properly). Mix well with fingers in order to get rid of any lumps of kuzu. Add the diluted kuzu to the pot, stirring constantly to avoid lumping.

As you stir, bring the mixture back to a boil (kuzu needs to boil in order to thicken). Let boil about 1 minute, as you continue stirring. It should become slightly thickened and a little glossy, like a gravy. Add the chopped strawberries and simmer 2 more minutes. Remove from heat and pour into serving cups. Let the kanten set for about 1 hour (refrigeration optional). Meanwhile, bring a pot of water to a boil. Drop the tofu in and let it cook for 2 minutes. Remove from water. Put the tofu, sweetener, vinegar, and vanilla in a blender or food processor. Whiz ingredients until smooth. Taste and adjust sweeteners to your liking. Chill until cool and a little thickened. When the kanten has set, garnish each serving with a dollop of the creamy tofu topping and top with a sprinkle of roasted almonds.

Variation

Use 5 heaping tablespoons of agar agar and eliminate the kuzu from the recipe. Let kanten set in a shallow pan. When it has gelled, put it in a blender with umeboshi vinegar and vanilla and blend until smooth. You may need to add a little apple juice to help it blend. Layer the blended kanten with the creamy topping to create a parfait.

nightshade vegetables

These are some of our culture's favorite foods: potatoes, tomatoes, peppers, and eggplant. Unfortunately for those who do most of their vegetable eating from this food group, they are very high in alkaloids, substances better associated with hallucinogens, medicines, and poisons. Nightshade vegetables are known for leeching calcium from the bones, and it is suspected that they contribute to its redistribution in the soft tissue of the body—resulting in kidney stones, arthritis, cancer, and a host of other problems. People on a health-recovery regimen are usually instructed to abstain from nightshades completely. Although I confess to eating french fries once in a while, most macrobiotic people I know rarely eat, or cook with, nightshades.

alcohol

I can't tell you how many people are blown away to find out that some macrobiotic people drink beer, sake, or whiskey on occasion. But these beverages are the result of grains being fermented, which is a natural process. And of course, the more natural the ingredients, the less sludgy the product.

Although alcohol is strong yin and not recommended for those trying to recover their health after serious illness, appropriate use of alcohol in moderation is not considered inherently bad. Let's put it this way: at a party, when the overall energy is expansive and connecting, I will drink a beer to go with the rhythm. I don't have to, but it feels nice and harmonizes with the overall energy taking place. Drinking in front of the TV alone because my life sucks, or getting plastered every night at a bar looking for Mister Wrong only makes everything worse.

If you have had an alcohol problem in the past, don't use this paragraph to justify picking up booze again. Often, it's much easier to just let go completely of the extremes that have enslaved us rather than manipulating a working relationship with them.

caffeine

I gotta be honest here: I love caffeine. Well, the first part of caffeine. It is a cheap, legal revved-up ego trip that gets my mind all excited about the future and all the Oscars I'm gonna win and what a *huge impact* I'm gonna have on the world. The second part of the caffeine trip sucks as badly as the first part is good; suddenly I'm scum, and so are you, and would you just learn how to drive or *get off the road!* It is one of the great examples of the yin and yang of everything. Because it is extreme, I don't use it regularly. And if the truth be told, I am much happier when it's not in my life at all.

CAFFEINE IS A PHYSICAL AND MENTAL STIMULANT

This is probably why most people use it. Coffee wakes up our bodies and minds. Its yin qualities drive energy up into the head and keep us on alert. But, because it is addictive, we start to need it to wake us up. This is especially true if your diet is heavy in rich and fatty foods. Stay away from caffeine for a week, eat whole grains, and after the headaches and lethargy subside, your energy will be much smoother and calmer. I try to use caffeine only when I feel that I really need it, when falling asleep at the wheel, for example, or in other extreme situations. The trouble is that, invariably, I want some more the next day. If you have any trouble sleeping, get rid of all caffeine products.

COFFEE AND OTHER CAFFEINE PRODUCTS CARRY SLUDGE

Coffee usually comes with all sorts of yucky and toxic pesticides. If you're going to drink coffee, make sure it's organic. Soda and diet drinks don't just carry sludge; they *are* sludge.

CAFFEINE GETS IN THE WAY OF THE UNIVERSE

When we're tense, overstimulated, and functioning mostly from our frontal lobes, a calm and clear connection to the Infinite Universe is hard to tap. Caffeine also overstimulates the adrenal glands and the heart, making us jumpy and talky. In this state, it becomes difficult to sit still and pick up our intuition.

CAFFEINE PRODUCES ANXIETY

Because caffeine activates your adrenal glands, your whole being gets the message that something is awry, like there's a lion chasing you across the kitchen. To be in this chronic state of alertness and defensiveness all the time can drain your body, mind, and soul quite completely. We are not meant to be dodging lions 24/7. Ex–caffeine drinkers are amazed when they realize how calm and peaceful life can be without their inner lion.

CAFFEINE LEECHES MINERALS

Like all the extreme foods, caffeine contributes to mineral loss. But here's a bonus: coffee is also very drying, so it *gives you wrinkles!*

CAFFEINE DOES OTHER BAD THINGS

For instance, it contributes to both female and male reproductive problems, breast cysts, gastrointestinal problems, cardiovascular stress, and nutritional deficiencies. Caffeine is not your friend.

genetically modified foods

Don't get me started: ugh. Too late. It makes me *crazy* that we have introduced freak foods into the public sector, without testing, without labeling, and we are dull and sleepy enough to think it won't have an impact. Since when do we know better how to evolve a species than nature does? This is pure arrogance, which Ohsawa said was the highest form of illness. What I do know is that pedigreed pets are the most neurotic. Dolly the cloned sheep had a host of physical problems. Eugenics didn't work for people, and it's not going to work for food.

It's one thing to be able to make a conscious choice between the factory-designed candy bar and a veggie burger. But these days, there is an 80 percent chance that the veggie burger contains genetically modified soybeans, and it has become increasingly difficult to make a choice aligned with nature. That really, really irks me. It bothers me that the decisions to label and test are made by people who don't seem to have much consciousness about what they eat and have no foresight about what they are creating. I hate that genetic engineering of foods has created patented foods, *owned* by the corporations who designed them. I *really* hate that genetically modified crops contaminate neighboring crops. Did you know that genetically modified foods can be designed with "suicide genes" that make their seeds useless, forcing the farmer to buy new seeds every year? What impact might that seedlessness, that lack of spark, have on us, energetically, over time? How is it that we expect to cross a fish with a strawberry and not affect our own genetic material? When was the last time you had sex with your gerbil?

And that's totally forgetting that genetically engineered crops can threaten natural biodiversity and the local food chains on agricultural land. A crop designed to resist herbicides means that so much herbicide can be used that there are no longer any weeds, which leaves nothing for the bugs, who die or go away, and there go the birds!

What I hate the most is that the impact of genetically modified foods will be slow, subtle, and probably untraceable within the matrix of crazy time bombs we have planted in our world. I want to cry when I think that these faceless mega-corporations will be able to argue in court, fifty years from now, that it was the cell phones, the air pollution, or the medication that caused the miscarriages or the undeveloped limbs or the gills of Jimmy the Fish Boy.

We are food. There is no separation. I trust nature, which has kept this planet spinning for billions of year, to design my food. Nature's genetic templates create natural people. Freaky templates create . . . ? We don't know yet. But do we really want to experiment on the entire world to find out? The whole thing makes a Big Mac look downright healthy.

It still makes sense to create a fuss about this. It's not too late to raise consciousness and e-mail your congressman about a thousand times to get him or her to support any legislation for GMO limits, labeling, and testing. Europeans are hopping mad about this stuff, and it makes it to the front pages of newspapers all the time. Greenpeace gets actively, creatively, and publicly angry, and I love that. Violations of the order of the universe this huge that affect so many people merit righteous, roiling anger. Yang repels yang.

Considering that GMOs have been in existence now for some time and that they have basically infiltrated the food chain, our only defense—on a physical level—is to eat as well as possible with what we know is natural and build bodies that can deal well with the altered foods that sneak in.

chemical preservatives and additives

This could be a very long passage, or a short one. I'll go for short: modern methods of food preservation and "enhancement" use chemicals and processes that are known to be unnatural, sludgy, and downright toxic. Ditto chemical additives. Because they are born of scientific manipulation, they have no natural life force, and inhibit or kill the energy of the foods. The worst part of these unpronounceables is that they are generally tasteless and colorless and we have gotten used to them. There are more than five thousand additives used in food production today. In terms of yin and yang, they include both extremes. They are probably, like GMOs, having a slow and steady impact on our well-being.

I hate being such a downer about the food supply, because life is about love and faith and not walking around pissed off and afraid of what we put in our mouths. That being said, joyfully choose organic foods with nature's energy intact, and your ability to feel good about life will be preserved and "enhanced."

the pill

Oral contraceptives keep your body hormonally "tricked" by juggling and manipulating the natural yin to yang to yin cycle of your femaleness, and therefore the reproductive energy that normally follows its own rhythm is thwarted. This level of intervention and manipulation can seriously impede your relationship to nature and skew your inner compass.

The pill can be very yang (which can lead to blood clots, stroke, or heart attack) or very yin and yang, depending on the combination of synthetic progesterone and estrogen used, but, regardless of the mix, it is definitely extreme.

The freedom to have sex whenever you want, without consciously considering pregnancy (or the avoidance of pregnancy), may seem like an important freedom, but is it being gained at the expense of other ones? You may want to investigate other, less invasive, forms of birth control in order to let your body find its own balance again.

recreational drugs

Generally, drugs are extreme and usually yin; they eventually (or quickly) lead to weakness, dullness, deterioration, and sometimes paranoia. I totally respect that the altered state of consciousness achieved through drugs can be mind expanding and pleasurable—at first. However, regular use of any kind of extreme, whether it's natural or synthetic, has serious consequences. Because drug use either sets your inner compass spinning wildly or inhibits your ability to read it, deep desludging of your body and consciousness cannot be achieved while using drugs.

CHAPTER SEVEN

phase three: going whole hog

So, you've decided to try to "go macro." Congratulations. You're gonna love it. By going whole hog, you are abstaining from the extreme foods that overtax the body. As you give your body a rest from the extremes and nourish it with moderate, balanced foods, the accumulated storage of sludge begins to dissolve and be discharged through normal channels. Old hardness and stagnation are released through urine, feces, or breath. Overly soft tissue regains its strength. Tightness becomes flexible. All extremes come back to center. Good-quality food strengthens the body and increases its natural capacity to protect itself. This is nature's medicine—unobstrusive, gentle, and just.

It is important to keep in mind that Phase Three is not an end point. I have not taken you this far to jam you down a narrow, one-way street. In fact, Phase Three can be incredibly exciting because it is can bring about such dramatic changes. It is in Phase Three that you do lots of desludging and refind your inner compass. Once it is buffed and polished, you can play freely, because you will have the tools and the intuition to bring yourself back to balance.

Some of the fruits of practicing Phase Three include lots of energy, clarity in thinking, renewed vitality, spiritual awakenings, mental flexibility, feeling younger, looking younger, connectedness with nature, emotional stability, inner peace, weight loss, beautiful skin, healthy hair, improved coordination, and much, much more. Phase Three, followed pretty well, is like opening a present from the universe every day. Try it for three months and see how you feel, but I urge you to consider committing to a clean macrobiotic practice for a year, because I believe that you will see a profound and dramatic shift in your whole approach to life.

In whole hog, you will let go of a few more foods, pick up a bunch of new ones, and step into a totally empowering and alchemical way of cooking. Going whole hog means becoming responsible for your own health and happiness. You are more powerful than you know.

your macrobiotic movie

I learned about the macrobiotic diet by looking at a pie chart that showed, by percentages, the amount of each category of food you should eat. But this model posed a few problems: first, people started putting food on their plates to look exactly like the pie chart (which made everything seem easy), but because the percentages were calculated by weight, not volume, they were eating too much of some things and not enough of others, day after day. But worse, the whole pie-chart image can be sort of restricting and dualistic, leading to worried thinking, like "Am I eating like a good, dutiful macro today, or did I go *outside the chart?!*" As if that were the worst thing that could ever happen and fling the eater out into the cold and lonely plains of "off the pie." The whole thing just makes me want to eat pie all the time!!

I tried to re-create the pie-chart model perfectly for a long time, and I finally had to surrender to my own needs—I do better with less grain, more vegetables, and more sweets. "Non Credo" of macrobiotics can mean "don't be a slave to concept" (see p. 17). Practicing macrobiotics is about recovering your freedom as a creation of the Infinite Universe, so there is *the* macrobiotic diet and then there is *your* macrobiotic diet, which will—of course—change.

So, given that I've watched the Oscars since I was seven, I have developed a system for all you movie lovers out there. I figure our lives are like our own personal movies, which we create daily. And in order to make a movie, you need a lot of different people and things, all playing very distinct and important roles.

Wherever pertinent, I have added how my movie model relates to the Standard Macrobiotic Diet as defined by Michio Kushi.

FOR BEST ACTOR IN A LEADING ROLE . . . THE OSCAR GOES TO . . . WHOLE-CEREAL GRAINS

Whole grains or whole-grain products are the leading men of your diet. They are your personal Tom Hanks, Harrison Ford, and Tom Cruise. Protagonists are solid and dependable, and the story generally revolves around them. They are strong and have limitless energy. Grains, like men, are more yang. More steadfast than flamboyant characters themselves, they make balance by seeking out mysterious, dynamic, sexy yin leading ladies, otherwise known as vegetables.

Your leading men include brown rice, barley, millet, quinoa, buckwheat, polenta, whole wheat, bulghur wheat, spelt, kamut, unyeasted sourdough bread, whole-wheat noodles, whole oats, rolled oats, and more.

Grains make up 50 to 60 percent of Michio Kushi's Standard Macrobiotic Diet.

FOR BEST ACTRESS IN A LEADING ROLE . . . VEGETABLES

What I love about vegetables is the variety that exists among them. Just as with women. Some are red, some are long, some are soft, some are fleshy, some are strong, some are graceful. Most have a mysterious and beautiful mix of many qualities. Vegetables keep us interested as a leading lady is supposed to. Think Halle Berry meets Lucy Liu meets Meryl Streep. Vegetables, being more yin than grains, bring this soft, interesting, dynamic energy to our plates and lives. And the dynamic charge between grains and vegetables is electric, like good chemistry on the screen. It is very common for people playing with macrobiotics to consider grain the principal food and get lazy with their vegetables. What they don't notice is that their movie is turning into a bad episode of *My Three Sons.*

Macrobiotic people try to stick to vegetables that occur naturally within their local climate, are organic whenever possible, and eaten within the season when they're grown. The theory is that if the earth can't produce it where you live, your body isn't getting what it needs to process it without some subtle stress and strain. Over time, that produces not-so-subtle stress and strain. On a daily basis, we try to incorporate the energies of upward, downward, and round vegetables to strike an overall balance in the body. Vegetables are either long-cooked or short-cooked, and both types are eaten every day. Potatoes, tomatoes, eggplant, and peppers—all members of the nightshade family of plants—are considered too extreme for regular use (see p. 162). Spinach and chard are also high in acids that leech minerals from the blood and bones, so take a pass on them.

In the Standard Macrobiotic Diet, Michio Kushi recommends 20 to 25 percent vegetables.

a note to women

When I first began macrobiotics, I ate "by the book," following the exact recommendations outlined in macro literature. And no matter where I looked, it said to eat 50 to 60 percent grain. So I did. What didn't occur to me at the time was that most of the dietary guidelines were designed by either Michio Kushi or George Ohsawa—both men—God bless 'em. While eating the food, I was also learning about yin and yang. More specifically, I was learning that men are governed by yang force and that women are governed by yin. So 50 to 60 percent grains (more yang) makes real sense for a male body and consciousness and probably feels really good to them. But one day, feeling particularly tight and moody, it *dawned* on me that, if men and women are governed by totally opposite forces, then maybe we should be eating totally opposite *foods,* in term of grains and vegetables. So I turned the Standard Diet on its head and starting eating 50 to 60 percent vegetables (more yin) and 20 to 25 percent grains (more yang). I immediately felt much looser, friendlier, and more feminine. Remember: *Non Credo.* It's easy to get "locked" on grain, both conceptually and physically. And yes, it should be eaten in order to get its amazing benefits. But macrobiotics is not about being perfect, or a slave, or an imitator; it's about being happy and free. It's good to follow guidelines in the beginning, in order to buff your inner compass, but after a while you should find out what makes *you* ridiculously happy. Don't be afraid to skip grain at a meal and see how you feel. Maybe today is a chick flick!

FOR BEST ACTRESS IN A SUPPORTING ROLE . . .
BEANS OR BEAN PRODUCTS

This is the character actress who rounds out the story. She keeps us laughing. She babysits the kids when the leading lady has to go on the car chase. She may be a little heavy, but we like her for that, because she represents solid, nurturing energy. She offers the advice, the information, the building blocks of the story when necessary. Think Kathy Bates or Frances McDormand. Without them, the movie is flimsy. The bean category includes aduki, kidney, split peas, garbanzos, black-eyed peas, lentils, soybeans, black soybeans, navy, great northern, anasazi, pinto, black turtle, and a variety of others. Bean products include tofu, tempeh, and natto soybeans.

The Standard Macrobiotic Diet recommends 10 percent beans or bean products a day. Personally, I just go for what is satisfying, which is probably about one cup a day.

FOR BEST SUPPORTING ACTOR . . .
SEA VEGETABLES

This is the old codger on the dock with the pipe and the fisherman's sweater. Maybe he's the protagonist's father, or a wise mentor. He is salty, like the sea. He is wise and through his pithy remarks keeps the whole story deep and meaningful. He gives us perspective and strength in wavering moments. He provides courage. These sea vegetables are hijiki, arame, wakame, kombu, nori, dulse, and agar agar. Sea vegetables show up subtly in most soups and bean dishes, but once a week this character comes to the fore for a nice strong arame or hijiki dish. It's also good to snack on half a sheet of nori every day.

The Standard Macro Diet recommends approximately 5 to 10 percent.

FOR BEST SOUND TRACK . . . SOUPS

Warm and fluid, soups soften and relax us like music. Soups can include grains, noodles, beans, fish, or simply vegtables. They are seasoned with sea salt, shoyu, or miso.

The Standard Macrobiotic Diet calls for 5 to 10 percent soups daily.

Simple miso soup is eaten almost every day. It's not unusual for macro people to have two bowls of soup a day.

FOR BEST COSTUMES . . . OCCASIONAL FOODS

Great clothes keep life interesting. These occasional foods "dress up" the diet. This category is dynamic because it includes strong yang (fish) and strong yin (sweeteners and fruit) for desserts. Of course, the best wardrobe is eclectic. Some macro people eat no fish at all, while others may partake three times a week. Just as your clothes present you to the world, it is the choices made in this category that can determine which way your energy leans vis-à-vis others. Big fish eaters have strong, active energy. Sweet lovers like me are more soft and reflective. Try on different foods like clothing to learn more and more about yin and yang.

This category, like your closet, includes a lot of different elements. They are:

- *Animal food:* usually fish, and mostly the white-fleshed variety (carp, red snapper, halibut, trout, haddock, flounder, cod, sole, and scrod). In the Standard Macrobiotic Diet, fish is suggested a few times a week for those in good health and is always served with some sort of fruit or dessert in order to balance its energy.
- *Fruits:* organic, local, in season, and often cooked. In a five-season climate, these include apples, apricots, cherries, grapes, peaches, pears, plums, tangerines, raisins or currants, blueberries, blackberries, raspberries, strawberries, cantaloupe, honeydew melon, and watermelon. In tropical climates, use tropical fruits. The Standard Diet recommends fruit a few times a week for those in good health.

- *Desserts:* made with natural sweeteners like barley malt, rice syrup, apple juice, and amazake. Occasionally maple syrup. Michio Kushi's Standard Diet suggests desserts two to three times a week.
- *Nuts:* these, too, are local and usually roasted, but not necessarily salted, since that's a good way to overeat both nuts and salt. Nut butters are much more difficult to digest than whole nuts and are used sparingly. Nontropical nuts include almonds, peanuts, walnuts, pecans, and chestnuts. Tropical nuts include brazil nuts, cashews, pistachios, and macadamias.
- *Seeds:* sesame seeds, pumpkin seeds, and sunflower seeds. The Standard Diet calls these "occasional snacks" and—together with nuts—are recommended not to exceed one to one-and-a-half cups a week for a healthy person.

FOR BEST DIRECTOR . . . SALT

Salt? Our Quentin Tarantino or John Ford? Salt is the director because we couldn't live without it. The proper amount of good-quality salt is totally necessary for life. The ocean is salty. Our blood is salty. Our tears are salty. Salt is the director because how you manage salt directs the rest of your choices. A little bit of salt has a big impact. Altering salt content is like the director giving one tiny direction that changes the entire course of the movie like, "Actually, Meryl, you are not a housewife, but a pro mud wrestler," and from then on, every scene she plays is completely different. The quality and amount of minerals in your diet determine how much protein you crave, which, in turn, determines your carbohydrate and fluid needs. When salt is out of whack, everything else is out of whack.

Salt is so powerful that too much of it can set up cravings for oil, sweets, fluids, and overeating. I learned this lesson the hard way, but after one too many binges, I began to moderate salt, and my compulsive eating habits were quelled substantially.

Salt is the most yang element of the film, bringing all the other forces together. An overbearing or controlling director (like too much salt) can leave you irritable and contracted, unable to flow creatively. Like a good director, salt should bring out the flavors of other foods, never dominating them. Salt remains behind-the-scenes, used in the kitchen, but never raw at the table.

The following seasonings, all with a salt component, are used most frequently in macrobiotic cooking:

- *Sea salt:* must be unrefined, preferably sun dried without chemicals to stop it from lumping. The current salt du jour in macrobiotics is a Mexican one called Si salt. Gray Celtic sea salt is considered too yang for daily use. In order to dissolve completely, sea salt (except in gomashio) should be cooked into the dish for at least ten minutes.
- *Miso* : this is one of life's most incredible foods. Miso is used in soups, condiments, and some vegetable dishes. As a fermented food, miso creates good-quality flora in the intestine. It also eliminates radioactive elements from the body. An overall blood purifier and alkalizer, miso soup is made almost every day. Miso needs to be simmered for two to three minutes but should not come to a boil, for that kills all its good enzymes.
- *Shoyu:* you will see this guy called "soy sauce" and "tamari" in older cookbooks. Technically, tamari is a by-product of miso making but has been confused with soy sauce for a long time. For our purposes, look for *shoyu,* which is the Japanese word for soy sauce and is what many health-food companies are naming their soy sauces. Check the label to make sure your shoyu contains no alcohol, which is used as a preservative for shoyu that has not been allowed to age sufficiently. Shoyu needs to be cooked into a dish for at least four minutes in order to break down properly.
- *Umeboshi plum and paste:* the umeboshi plum is right up there with miso as an incredible food. This small, reddish plum, pickled with salt and shiso leaves, is both salty and sour and packs a serious wallop. It is used to cook grain but also as a seasoning in dressings. Umeboshi plums are also just eaten as a pickle with grain. It is a basic ingredient in the most common home remedies because umeboshi plums alkalize the blood so effectively. Great for nausea, heartburn, hangovers, diarrhea, and a host of other things.

- *Condiments,* which include gomashio, tekka, pumpkin shiso, shio kombu, nori flakes, and many more: they are very good for mineralizing and alkalizing the blood but should be used sparingly, since they are mostly salty in taste (about one teaspoon of gomashio a day and a sprinkle of the others). Men, governed by yang energy, can get away with a little more than women can.

FOR BEST PICKLES . . . PICKLES

I couldn't think of a movie counterpart to pickles. Can you? Pickles are used in your macrobiotic movie to help you digest other foods, grains in particular. Pickles promote salivation and have good-quality enzymes that help break down food and provide strong energy. Whether it's pickled herring, tempeh, yogurt, or an olive, every culture eats some kind of fermented food. Salty or store-bought pickles should be rinsed or soaked to make them milder. Approximately one tablespoon of pickle is eaten every day, usually with grain.

FOR BEST LIGHTING . . . GARNISHES

Garnishes literally "lighten" the energy of dishes, bringing a fresh, upward yin component to a warm, hearty dish. Like good lighting, they open up a subtle energetic and artistic dimension to cooking as they add taste, color, and panache. Garnishes are used on all soups, some vegetable dishes, and any other place you see fit. They include scallions, parsley, cilantro, lemon wedges, nori strips, chives, radishes, and carrot florets or anything nice you can think up.

FOR AFTER THE SHOW . . . BEVERAGES

Beverages are consumed after a meal, as opposed to during. In fact, unlike most folks, macrobiotic people don't chug down liquid just because it is recommended; as I mentioned earlier, that recommendation is aimed at a nation with meat as its principal food. Plus, too much water is like too much of anything—an extreme that can create imbalances and overtax the kidneys. With a grain-and-vegetable-based diet, which is naturally rich in fluid, these excesses don't occur, and there is no reason to force the kidneys to do so much work. We drink when we're thirsty, and the choices include spring or well water, and teas such as kukicha, bancha, roasted rice, and barley. There is even a tea called "Mu 16" that George Ohsawa formulated from sixteen different herbs. Less frequently (like a few times a week), carrot juice, celery juice, apple juice, amasake, and grain coffee. Beer and sake are there for people in good health. Generally avoided during desludging are strongly aromatic teas, carbonated drinks, ice-cold beverages, soy milk, soda pop, coffee, and hard liquor. You will meet, as you explore the macrobiotic world, people who drink actual coffee on a regular basis, proving that nobody's perfect—thank God.

EXTRAS . . . OCCASIONAL SEASONINGS

Occasional seasonings include lemon, brown rice vinegar, umeboshi vinegar, mirin (cooking wine made from rice), garlic, horseradish, and ginger. I kind of have a thing for ume vinegar, and I use it in desserts to bring out the sweet flavor. Most aromatic herbs and spices are avoided for desludging but can be used in moderation by healthy people. Oils used in regular cooking are sesame and toasted sesame. Less frequently used (although I use them a lot) are olive, corn, safflower, and sunflower oils. All oils, whenever possible, are unrefined.

WORDS OF ADVICE

Buy organic grains, beans, and produce whenever possible. Pesticides are sludge. And luckily it is getting easier and easier to find these groovy foods all over the place. Although I have a policy of avoiding putting anything that ends with the suffix "cide"—which means "murder"—in my body, it's impossible to do it 100 percent. And if variety in your diet is severely limited by the nonavailability of organic foods, it's better to have some nonorganic variety than to go crazy about being strictly pesticide-free. Eating just rice, broccoli, and carrots for months on end is not okay, because such fare lacks variety and will eventually create imbalances. Keep in mind that this whole thing is about freedom, not perfection, and variety is actually an expression of good-quality yin force.

If you're facing a serious health challenge and have the money, you might consider ordering organic produce online and having it shipped to you. See Resources at the back of the book for more details.

kitchen setup

Remember Sea Monkeys? I got some when I was about eight and I was *so excited* about them that, long before reading the instructions, I dumped the Sea Monkey powder into the water and watched, with bated breath. Of course, nothing happened. I hadn't read that I was supposed to put the special magic *preparation* solution in the water first and then wait an excruciating and quite impossible twenty-four hours before dumping in the monkey dust.

That's my way of saying that I've never liked cookbooks that make you think you have to have the perfect macro kitchen before you can do a thing. I hope you're excited about macrobiotic cooking, and I don't want anything to hold you back. Chances are you've been cooking a little (or a lot) already and have done a great job. The following are implements that will make your whole-foods cooking even more delicious and beautiful.

THE ESSENTIALS

Sharp knife—eventually a heavy Japanese vegetable knife is best
Heavy pot with a heavy lid, preferably enameled cast iron
Flame deflector or flame tamer, available at any cooking store
Stainless-steel skillet and a couple of stainless-steel pots

That's it. The rest, for now, you can fudge.

I'm Assuming You Already Have
Blender
Strainer

Colander

Mixing bowls

Baking sheet

Wooden spoons

Slotted spoons

Steamer basket or bamboo steamer

You Might As Well Chuck

The microwave oven

Teflon or aluminum cookware

Down the Road Apiece

Gas stove (or small propane stove)

Wooden cutting board

Stainless-steel pressure cooker

Wooden rice paddles

Cast-iron skillet

You Know You're Really Macro When You Own

Sushi mats

Chopsticks

Suribachi and surikogi

Juicer

Hand food mill

Ohsawa pot

Nabe pot

Pickle press

A picture of George Ohsawa hanging in your kitchen!

Stock Your Cupboard with

A variety of beans, dried

Canned organic beans

A variety of grains

Dried sea vegetables

Whole-wheat bread and pastry flour

Olive, corn, and sesame oil

Safflower oil for deep frying

Shoyu

Miso

Sea salt

Umeboshi vinegar

Brown rice vinegar

Mirin (rice wine for cooking)

A variety of noodles

Sweeteners: rice syrup, barley malt, maple syrup

Fresh tofu

Dried tofu

A variety of snacks from the health-food store

Tempeh

Whole-wheat pita bread

Whole-wheat tortillas

Puffed rice

Crispy rice for Crispy Rice Treats

Organic apple juice

Amasake

Bottled carrot juice, or carrots and a juicer

Agar agar

Kuzu

Frozen fruit for kantens in winter

Dried fruit

Roasted seeds and nuts

Raw vegetables to snack on

Good-quality dips, made of tofu, beans, etc.

Store-bought hummus

Polenta, even premade

Rolled oats

Mochi

Organic popcorn

All-fruit jams

Fruit spritzers

ABUNDANCE

I encourage you to have all this stuff on hand, in abundance, because it will help you to not feel deprived. You are making a move that, although it's becoming more popular all the time, with respect to the world of 7-Elevens, normal grocery stores, and gas-station checkout counters, goes severely against the grain. All it takes is one Kit Kat bar staring me in the face after I've pumped my gas on a brutally cold day to make my chin quiver like that of a little girl left behind on the class trip. My whole macro world seems so ridiculous and stupid at that moment, so small and dark and lonely. The Kit Kat looks so happy, so free and easy in the world, loved by everyone.

Yes, this is neurotic. But it's also an expression of energy law. The bright and flashy world of convenience food DOES move faster, have more dates, and carry more superficial charge than the rice in your kitchen. It is more dangerous and exciting in an "I'm gonna go home with you tonight and make sweet love to you and then I'll never, ever return your phone calls and make you feel insane while you crave me, desperately, for weeks" kind of way. Familiar? These feelings of grief and change and isolation are real. So it's crucial, at that moment, that I have my own rice-syrup-sweetened Rice Crispy Treat either in my freezing pocket or in my freezing car. Because then the little kid inside me feels okay. And until that little girl feels comfortable in the health-food store and really digs her ice-cream substitute, she must be treated with serious TLC.

cooking for noncooks

If you are someone who is attracted to this information for philosophical or health reasons but are not exactly a kitchen goddess, I can relate. There's nothing worse than someone waxing erotic about vegetables and cast-iron frying pans to make me want to go to see a movie. But I have learned over the years that cooking has its benefits.

When I cook for myself, I am in the driver's seat of my life. I am no longer being pushed around by the forces of the day, other people's moods, a Snickers bar, or Burger King. Having chopped and stewed, simmered and blanched, then eating all the energy I have put out, I am declaring to myself, in the most concrete way possible, that I am on my side. I love myself inasmuch as love is attention and touching and care. We look very hard in therapy and self-help books for that magical clue to self-love. Let's look inside the pressure cooker.

When you cook for yourself, you have power in your own life. Period. And we all want more power in our own lives. So don't cook because it's fun, or because it's "good for you," or because you're a good wife or girlfriend. Cook because you are greedy, selfish, and conniving. Yay!

meal planning: achieving balance

A confession: it took me FOREVER to understand what *macros* meant by "balance." So let me save you some time and grief:

- Is "balance" equal parts yin to equal parts yang? Not when it comes to food for humans. That's a big one, and it took me a long time to get up the guts to ask that question. As humans, we receive about 5 to 7 parts heaven's force (yang) to 1 part earth's force (yin). Think about it: if the earth's force were stronger, we'd fly off the planet! So our food should be the opposite: about 5 to 7 parts earth's force to 1 part heaven's force in order to feel bouncy and happy in our bodies.
- Don't think about those ratios too much. You can go crazy trying to balance perfectly, and the numbers don't really matter in the kitchen.
- As long as you are choosing macrobiotic quality foods (without going crazy on the salt and seasonings, which will make you too yang), you should be in the right range. Experiment and continually discover what feels right for you.
- Balance is a different for every person. Only you know what makes you feel happy and free.
- Balance changes all the time; what works to achieve balance in the summer doesn't necessarily work in the winter.
- When people refer to a "balanced meal," they mean a meal that contains the basic components for the average person to feel nourished and

satisfied. Some meals are simple and some are complicated. A fully fleshed-out balanced meal, with all the bells and whistles includes:

- A soup
- A grain dish
- A bean, bean product, or fish dish
- A long-cooked vegetable
- A short-cooked vegetable
- A sea-vegetable dish (included a few times a week)
- A pickle
- A condiment
- A dessert (a few times a week)
- A postmeal beverage

Keep in mind that no one—in good health—needs to cook this much every day, let alone every meal. I present you with this model because it is the complete picture of all the macrobiotic components for restoring balance and supporting your health, but you don't need to have all these components at every meal in order to desludge and stay healthy (see examples of balanced meals on pp. 163–165).

I recommend that you eventually aim at cooking a meal like the one above a few times a week, but don't get freaked out if it takes a while—maybe months—for you to achieve that. This is not a race, and no one is watching you. If all you can manage now is brown rice and steamed broccoli, that's perfect. Just chew well and feel proud of yourself.

Know that from a fully fleshed-out, balanced meal you can use leftovers of grain, bean, long-cooked vegetable, sea vegetable, pickle, and dessert for meals the next day (see Leftovers, p. 174).

The "balancing" that a macrobiotic cook does in the kitchen consists of playing with different sets of complementary opposites. Through the choices she makes, she alters the character of the meal, and the impact it will have on the body. The sets of opposites include:

- Grains and vegetables
- Grains and beans

- Downward- and upward-growing vegetables
- Land vegetable and sea vegetable
- Dry and wet
- Hard and soft
- Heavy and light
- Hot and cool
- Cooked and raw
- Strongly seasoned and lightly or unseasoned
- Animal food and fruit
- Long cooked and short cooked

She also plays with colors: red, orange, yellow, green, brown, black, and white, including as many as she can. And she chooses from the spectrum of tastes: sweet, bitter, sour, salty, and pungent, hoping to include them all in a day, or even a meal.

So begin to play with these puzzle pieces in the kitchen, no matter your culinary prowess: where there is grain, add some vegetable. If you have a dry piece of bread, spread it with some moist hummus. Balance a downward carrot with an upward celery stick. Where there is a heavy bean dish, add a garnish of raw, upward scallion. As you desludge, you will become more sensitive to what "balance" means to you. Eventually, you will have a lot of fun and creative satisfaction as you intuitively make each meal a dynamic expression of yin and yang. Here are some examples of "balanced meals."

A Healing Balanced Meal
   Miso soup
   Rice with barley
   Aduki beans with squash and kombu
   Nishime vegetables
   Steamed greens
   Pickled red radish
   Gomashio
   Strawberry kanten with creamy topping
   Kukicha tea

A One-Pot Balanced Meal
Barley stew with lentils, wakame, carrots, onions, and celery
Bancha tea

A Simple Balanced Meal
Scrambled tofu with carrots, burdock, onions, and corn
Rice with umeboshi plum
Blanched greens
Barley tea

A Quick Balanced Meal
Leftover steamed sourdough bread
Leftover hummus
Leftover homemade pickles
Fresh salad
Cool kukicha tea

A Relaxing Balanced Meal
Nabe vegetables with tofu
Rice with barley
Ginger pickle
Warm apple juice

A Strengthening Balanced Meal
Miso soup with ginger
Fried seitan with gravy
Pressure-cooked rice with sauerkraut
Kinpira
Boiled salad
Kukicha tea

An Elegant Balanced Meal
Light miso soup
Filet of sole with grated daikon
Elegant Orange Couscous
Arame with onions and corn

Fresh salad with mustard umeboshi dressing
Amasake pudding
Beer

A Balanced Thanksgiving Meal
Carrot Soup
Tofu turkey with seitan stuffing and mushroom gravy
Long-grain rice with wild rice, apples, and raisins
Corn bread
Boiled salad with pumpkin-seed dressing
Pumpkin pie with Vanilla Rice Dream
Grain coffee

your cooking plan

When I first looked at menus that included six or seven dishes for one meal, I was totally overwhelmed and intimidated. But remember when you first learned to drive a car, just cruising down the street was terrifying, and now you drive a stick, talk on the cell phone, eat a muffin, and check out the guy walking down the street—all at the same time!! For now, all you need to do is start with grains and vegetables. Make that your beginning. Like just driving the car. As you master some grain dishes and some yummy vegetables dishes, you'll naturally be ready for more.

Although it has become normal for me to cook complicated meals, I still feel uncomfortable approaching it without a plan. Having a decent plan makes cooking *ten thousand times* more serene. So before you pick up a knife, pick up a pen and plan your meal like this:

MAKE A LIST OF THE DISHES

- Rewrite the list according to estimated cooking time, longest to shortest.
- Now write down, beside each dish, the major movements of each dish— e.g., beans: soaking, pressure-cooking, seasoning OR grain, washing,

boiling, seasoning, simmering OR soup: chopping vegetables, boiling, seasoning, garnishing. This forces your subconscious mind to think through the movements of every dish. This is very important, because you are literally "practicing" all the actions in your mind. Then the doing of them becomes much smoother, with no surprises.

• Now look over all the movements and start to see what needs to happen first. Then second, etc. Put a number next to each movement, showing yourself where to go next. Keep in mind that cooking is never a straight line; it is always a spiral. One dish needs some sort of attention, and then, while it moves to its next stage, you bring your awareness to another dish. You keep moving, going back and forth between dishes, like helping your kids get ready to go to school on a winter day. You may not be absolutely correct in the order of each movement, but it doesn't matter. The point is that you have thought it through and that you have a list to refer to if you get lost.

• Once you have plotted out all the movements, put your plan somewhere dry and visible and begin with action number 1.

SET A TIMER

A timer creates a sacred space. And I don't mean sacred like woo-woo, waa-waa women dancing under a full moon on a hilltop, although I've done that and, provided the weather cooperates, it's sort of fun. I mean sacred like apart, defined, different.

I need a defined slot of time in the kitchen because sometimes when I am cooking, I can get this female martyr voice in my head, which I fantasize that I share with my sisters everywhere; it says to me, as I thrust the steel wool across the greasy baked-on residue: "This is the horrible indentured servitude that women have suffered for millennia. Gloria Steinem doesn't do this. You are a slave. Nothing has changed." Funnily enough, these thoughts don't help. Nor do "I hate this" or "This is gonna take forever." They make cooking a sort of . . . heavy and negative experience. When I set the timer, I feel lighter and freer and imagine myself a Tibetan monk gleefully sweeping out the monastery.

So use an egg timer. Or use the timer on your stove. But watching the clock won't do. I repeat: watching the clock is not the same thing. Because then, on some level, you are stressing out about watching the clock. The point here is to *relieve* you of stress instead of adding to it.

As you begin cooking macrobiotically, you will want to put sixty minutes on the timer, because beans and grains will take about an hour. Then while they cook, you do everything else. While the timer is ticking, you pay attention to what you are doing. Maybe you've got a little music playing, but that's it. You let the machine pick up the phone. Let your partner or a video engage the kids. You commit fully to the tasks at hand. You experiment, you problem-solve, you discover things like a kid in science class. And when that blessed timer beeps, you wrap things up and stop. You leave the kitchen and live the rest of your day to the fullest. Cooking is over. Maybe there is no garnish for the soup. Perhaps you never made it to the seaweed dish. Who cares? It doesn't matter. The Macro Police are over at Madonna's house. Plus, your sanity and happiness are much more important than having a perfectly balanced meal every day.

Finally, you are on a learning curve; as you continue, you will get more and more done within an hour, because practice always makes better. By the way, it doesn't need to be sixty minutes every day. In fact, it may be more like sixty one day and forty-five the next, because beans, which take the longest to cook, only need to be made every other day. With good planning, your time can be used very effectively.

SAY A PRAYER

When in doubt, ask the universe for help. It's important that you begin to see cooking for what it truly is: the propeller of your entire life, from your cells up. You might want to post the following prayer in order to remember that your mind-blowing superpowers are crouching latent in the pilot light of your stove.

Dear Infinite Universe:
I am a magician.
Through the alchemy of cooking,
I am turning this time into glittering gold.
I am building my body

And the bodies of those I love.

Instead of stagnation,

I am enjoying growth and forward motion.

Instead of hiding my light, it is glowing in the world.

It feels so good to be alive.

Cooking wakes up my senses,

Sharpens my intuition,

And warms my soul.

Cooking is cool.

Thank you for teaching me, through cooking

About your elements;

Fire, earth, metal, water, and tree

Which make up my body and all living things.

With you,

I am nourishing my deepest power

And my wildest dreams.

Let's go!

leftovers

Because all this cooking takes time and energy, make sure you always make enough food for the next day. Macrobiotics is all about the life force of food, which diminishes rather quickly, so we do not keep foods as leftovers for long periods of time. Too often, I have heard people say that they make one big pot of rice and just eat from it for the entire week. It sounds so easy, but there is very little oomph left in the rice by Thursday. And yes, rice is better for you than a bowl of ice cream—even rice that's four days old—but it's much better for your overall condition to take the time to make new stuff. I realize that nobody's perfect on this, but my point is to discourage you from eating really old leftovers as a habit.

Another annoying fact: we don't generally freeze things, because not only is the original energy depleted by the cold, but the molecular structure of food changes after freezing.

Here's what to know in terms of how long each food lasts, from longest to shortest:

- *Condiments:* dry condiments (like gomashio) last one to two weeks. Wet condiments (like nori) last about a week, refrigerated.
- *Pickles:* last about a week.
- *Most desserts:* use within a few days.
- *Bean dishes:* use within forty-eight hours of cooking.
- *Grain dishes:* use within twenty-four hours of cooking.
- *Soups:* use within twenty-four hours of cooking (except miso soup).
- *Long-cooked vegetable dishes:* use within twenty-four hours of cooking.
- *Sea-vegetable dishes:* use within twenty-four hours of cooking.
- *Pressed salads:* use within twenty-four hours of making.
- *Short-cooked vegetable dishes:* make fresh daily.
- *Miso soup:* make fresh daily.

Given the above, you will be eating lots of the dishes you make the next day. It is best, if you have the time and inclination, to get creative with your leftovers. Here are some ideas:

- Fry up leftover grain with some vegetables.
- Make bean soup into an aspic, using agar agar.
- Reheat whatever you can (eating cold food makes you cold inside) but if the microwave's your only option at work, then skip it.
- Combine dishes whenever possible to make them into something totally new. For instance, combine a pressed salad with cooked grain to make a light grain salad.
- Roll some pressed salad into a cooked collard green to make a green roll.
- Form leftover grain or beans (or a combination) into patties and fry them up. Make a dipping sauce.

If these suggestions sound overwhelming right now, just forget about them. Take your time and keep it simple. I don't want you freaking out over being the perfect macro person. As you get more adept at cooking, making creative choices will feel more and more natural.

a typical macro day

Wake up with the sun.
Feel sublime.
Be thankful for every single blade of grass that has ever been grown under
  the sun.
Chew rice four thousand times.
Plant new rice in backyard rice paddy.
Make homemade clothes for twelve children.
Homeschool the children.
Smile.
Appreciate life.
Cook nineteen-course meal.
Chew rice nine thousand times.
Harvest rice.
Write letters to loved ones around the world, thanking them for just being.
Call Gwyneth and gossip.
Put twelve children to bed.
Make love to soul mate.
ZZZZZzzz.

Actually, I have no freakin' clue what other macrobiotic people do all day, but here's a glimpse at what they might eat:

- *Breakfast:* leftover grain (usually cooked soft to make a porridge), greens. Maybe some roasted seeds, or rice syrup. It is not uncommon to have miso soup at breakfast.
- *Lunch:* leftovers from the night before, sometimes livened up, sometimes not, plus a lightly cooked green vegetable.
- *Snack:* leftovers or carrot juice, apple juice, popcorn. Possibly a dessert from the day before.

- *Dinner:* a freshly cooked balanced meal, creating leftovers for the next day.

Of course, whatever keeps you nourished and happy is what's right for you. But with just an hour in the kitchen every day, you can work some serious magic.

eating out

Don't think that just because you're macro, you gotta hang out at home all the time. Living without dairy, white sugar, and most meats is not as hard as you might think. These days, there are lots of options for eating out.

If you live in a big city, there are probably some good health-food restaurants. Check them out. My one caution is to not compare your cooking to restaurant cooking because restaurants generally use much more salt than you should in the kitchen. Remember that salt is the director of your movie, and a light hand is key.

- *Mexican:* try a cheeseless burrito, or a big Mexican salad, hold the cheese. Corn chips and guacamole.
- *Japanese:* sushi, tempura, dumplings, miso soup, salads, and more. But you should know that sushi rice has sugar in it and that the shoyu you're dipping it into is very salty. If you want to get around that, ask for sushi made with "kitchen rice" and either use the mild soy sauce or bring a dilution of your own. If you want to get really anal (I have), bring your own pickled ginger, either unsweetened or sweetened with natural sweeteners. Don't depend on miso soup at Japanese restaurants to serve as your daily, desludging miso—theirs is yummy, but it may contain MSG, less-than-stellar-quality miso, and is most likely overcooked.
- *Chinese:* I try to go to places that don't use MSG. And then I ask whether a dish has sugar in it. Stuff can generally be made without sugar if you ask. Lots of great vegetable and fish dishes to enjoy.
- *Thai:* again, sugar, salt, and MSG are the big issues here. I have yet to find a place that won't make pad thai without sugar.

- *Italian:* fish, pasta, vegetables. Yum. Italian food tends to go heavy on the nightshade vegetables and cheese, but when I feel like breaking the mold with a nice tomato sauce over noodles, there's no place like a good Italian joint. There is probably sugar in most tomato sauces, so if you're looking to really avoid that, ask or avoid it altogether. Get noodles with garlic and olive oil.
- *Fancy restaurants:* when I have to go into the regular world, socially or on business, and I don't have any control over where we eat, I tend to stick with fish, vegetables, and some sort of grain product, like white rice or noodles. Most restaurants will serve a decent side of vegetables, a good salad, and it is in these situations that, if nothing else satisfies, I eat potatoes.

Life is about play. So enjoy everything to the hilt. But I trust you understand that eating out day after day, is not supportive of your freedom, over time. With someone else always making the decisions about what goes in you, and therefore deciding who you are, your power over your own reality is reduced. At the same time, life sucks if you feel chained to the stove. So enjoy eating out for what it is—a change in energy, a break from the kitchen, socializing, being pampered, new tastes—but do it in moderation.

If you have seen a counselor and are using macrobiotics in order to recover from a medical condition, follow your counselor's directions regarding restaurant eating.

macrograduate school: yangizing and yinnizing

Once you've gotten used to working with your inner compass—in life and in the kitchen—it's important that you know how to make dishes more yin and how to make them more yang. By adjusting your cooking to harmonize with the season, the day, or your mood, you can cook to truly support your body and soul. In this section, I have listed what you can do in the kitchen to pull a dish in either the yin or yang direction. Then I have included possible menus for each season. Try them out, but let them be springboards for your own imagination.

THINGS TO DO IF YOU ARE FEELING WEAK OR SCATTERED (YIN) AND WANT TO FEEL MORE CENTERED AND STRONG (YANG)

- Make long-cooking dishes that warm and stabilize the body
- Add a tiny bit more salt or seasoning to dishes
- Use ¼ to ½ umeboshi plum as your pickle
- Make a sea-vegetable dish like arame or hijiki
- Apply a little pressure by pressure-cooking grains or pressing a salad
- Make soups heartier with chunkier vegetables and less water
- Make sure you include root vegetables in the meal (but don't skip the greens!)
- Avoid strong spices

More yang choices are made in the later summer, autumn, and winter. Here are some sample menus:

A Late Summer Menu
  Squash soup
  Millet "potatoes" with kuzu gravy
  Arame with onions
  Mock tuna
  Boiled greens
  Pickled red radishes
  Crispy rice treats
  Kukicha tea

An Autumn Menu
  Miso soup
  Pressure-cooked brown rice with chestnuts
  Aduki beans with kombu and squash

Nabe vegetables with dip sauce

Daikon pickle

Baked pears with pecan cream

Kukicha tea

A Winter Menu

Split Pea Soup

Kasha with sauerkraut

Tempura vegetables and tofu with grated daikon

Fresh salad

Apple crisp

Mu tea

THINGS TO DO IF YOU FEEL STRESSED, IRRITABLE, OR PRESSURED (YANG) AND WANT TO FEEL MORE RELAXED (YIN)

• Reduce or avoid salty seasonings and condiments

• Rinse or soak your pickles well to reduce saltiness

• Include much more vegetable than grain in the meal

• Emphasize green and upward-growing vegetables

• Make soups more watery, with vegetables cut in smaller pieces

• Emphasize short-cooking methods

• Have a dessert (but not a baked one, as baking is very yang)

• Eliminate pressure-cooking and reduce pressing time for salads

• Use some sweetener or fruit in cooking

More yin choices are made in the spring and summer. Here are some sample menus:

A Springtime Menu

Lentil soup

Mediterranean barley salad

Boiled salad with lots of leafy greens

Strawberry kanten with tofu cream
Barley tea

A Summer Menu
Corn soup
Quinoa salad or tabbouleh (both contain pickles)
Hummus with kayu bread
Stir-fried vegetables
Watermelon
Cool kukicha tea

BUT KEEP IN MIND . . .

It's easy to look at the above categories and think, "Okay. I'll just have salty, deep-fried carrots all winter and then change to steamed celery in the spring. That'll do me." But it's not that simple. Through cooking, we want to harmonize with the seasons, helping our bodies to adjust to the changes, so that means we emphasize certain foods and cooking styles in each season. However, because nothing is entirely yin or entirely yang, there is always a little bit of the opposite in every season, and it is important to choose from all the energies on a daily basis in order to stay truly in touch with the mysterious, dynamic life force. So a meal in April should have more greens and lighter cooking than other elements, but it also needs to be grounded by some roots vegetables, too. Think of it this way: when you were a kid and it was your birthday, you were celebrated, given gifts and lots of love—but that didn't mean that your parents kicked your siblings out of the house; everyone understood that they were valuable members of the family, simply not celebrated in quite the same way that day. Soon enough, they would have birthdays, too, when the roles would be reversed.

At the peaks of the energy shifts, the summer and winter solstices, the energy is so extreme that you may crave its opposite. For instance, people get oranges in their stockings at Christmas and eat deep-fried fish 'n' chips in July. Go with what your body tells you, because life is one big paradox.

macrobiotic lifestyle suggestions

As if I haven't told you enough new stuff to do, here's a little more. Because we are concerned with getting "up close and personal" with the Infinite Universe, it is important to consider all the ways (besides food) we invite this healing energy in, or shut it out. I recommend, unless you are in a healing crisis and need to make major changes quickly, that you try a few of these on for size, or go one at a time—it's important that you recognize their effects on you in order to really integrate them into your life.

THE BODY SCRUB

This is an excellent and addictive picker-upper. Forget your coffee in the morning; a daily body scrub will awaken all the meridians of your body and your internal organs and get you revved up for your day, without any downside. Here's how it's done:

- Fill your sink with hot, hot water.
- Dunk a washcloth in it and let it soak a few seconds. Remove the washcloth and wring it out.
- Fold it twice so that it's one quarter its original size and the heat stays in it longer.
- With this wet, hot little rectangle, scrub your face (avoiding your eyes), applying enough pressure to turn the skin pink. Don't forget the back of your neck, your ears, etc. Redunk the washcloth and repeat the scrubbing on your chest, armpits, down the arms, redunking whenever the washcloth cools off. Scrub until the skin turns pink. Parts of you may be blotchy pink, but don't worry. Over time, they will even out.
- Be sure to do your hands and every finger. Scrub your back, your belly, and your groin area, but avoid your privates. The armpits and the groin area are home to many lymph nodes, and scrubbing there helps to move lymph fluid, which strengthens immunity. Go down the legs, getting your ankles, the bottoms of your feet, and every toe. Yowza!

The whole body scrub should take about five to ten minutes, depending upon your attentiveness to detail, and will feel AMAZING. When you don't have lots of time, just do your face, hands, and feet for a major wake-up call. The body scrub can be done morning and night, although I just do it upon waking. This scrubbing increases circulation, sloughs off old skin, and helps to break down energy sludge that's getting in between you and the Infinite Universe.

AVOID EATING THREE HOURS BEFORE GOING TO BED

In other words, go to bed on an empty stomach. You see, sleep is for recharging your body. It is the time when the Infinite Universe does lots of secret work on you—like a CIA agent—and the emptier you are of material food, the more you can receive vibrational food. This is very important in terms of getting rest, losing weight, and discharging sludge. If you have eaten anything before going to bed, your intestines, liver, and kidneys spend the whole night working instead of resting. If you have a hard time waking up in the morning, follow this suggestion religiously for a little while (along with the body scrub) and you will be amazed at the change in your A.M. humor.

DRINK ONLY WHEN YOU'RE THIRSTY

There is no other bodily mechanism that we disrespect quite like thirst. We eat when we're hungry (or have low blood sugar), we pee when we get the signal that our bladder is full, we have sex when we're horny, we sleep when we're tired, and yet we think we know better than thirst. Dousing yourself with fluid all day every day is not benign. Try dousing your plants with water and see how they do. Water is an extremely powerful element that can erode rocks over time. Yes, we are mostly fluid, but we are also home to other energies, like the complex workings of our stomach, spleen, and pancreas, and the fire of our small intestine. The term *fire in the belly* refers to a natural, digestive fire in us that needs to stay stoked in order to maintain a healthy life. When we douse ourselves with water—especially cold water—it dilutes digestive enzymes, overworks the kidneys, and dampens our inner fire. The mechanism of thirst is our barometer for keeping our fluids balanced. As it should be. Respect it. Finally, the macrobiotic diet is so fluid-rich already that you will do much less water chugging than you feel the need to when you're eating a meat, sugar, and bread diet. If you do find that you are thirsty all the time, reduce your salt intake.

AVOID LONG HOT BATHS AND SHOWERS

By long I mean, more than fifteen or twenty minutes. After about twenty minutes of exposure to hot water, the body begins to release minerals, and if you make long showers or baths a regular practice, you can become demineralized and weak.

USE NATURAL BODY PRODUCTS

Think of it this way—your skin is the largest organ of your body, and it literally sucks stuff in. So when I am buying a skin-care product, I read the label and ask myself if I would be comfortable drinking the ingredients, because slathering them on my body is almost the same thing. Just about everything you need comes in a healther version, and even foods can do the trick—e.g., sesame or peanut oil as moisturizer, oatmeal as a facial pack. Christina Pirello has written a great book called *Glow* all about this. Check it out.

USE SHEETS, TOWELS, BLANKETS, RUGS, AND CLOTHES MADE OF NATURAL MATERIALS

This means cotton, silk, linen, and wool. If you have the luxury of building your own home, do your best to choose natural materials throughout. Natural materials still contain natural energy, and more important, don't block energy as synthetic materials can. Just think of how much you sweat when you're wearing polyester—energy can't get out! If we are looking to harmonize with nature and let the Infinite Universe in, it's important to surround ourselves with natural vibes.

KEEP FRESH PLANTS IN THE HOME

Not only pretty but also energizing, plants enliven any atmosphere.

OPEN WINDOWS TO CIRCULATE FRESH AIR, EVEN IN WINTER

Even if it's just thirty minutes a day, fresh air in the home is vital to your health. In summer, use fans instead of air-conditioning. This may sound crazy now, but after you have not eaten sugar, dairy, and lots of meat for a while, you will not suffer in warm weather because your internal air-conditioning will function again.

MINIMIZE THE USE OF ELECTRICAL MACHINERY CLOSE TO THE BODY

Cell phones, hair dryers, and electric toothbrushes create really intense vibes that are a million miles from natural. Overexposure to nonorganic energy sources can affect your organic energy system in a negative way over time.

THROW OUT THE MICROWAVE

Sorry. I'll admit it's convenient, but you gotta admit it's creepy. Nature can't cook bacon that way, so you shouldn't, either. The electromagnetic radiation necessary for microwave cooking is so intense and so yin (whereas normal heat comes from yang energy) that it is weakening to the blood and produces chaotic energy. Don't let yourself be a guinea pig in the mass microwave experiment taking place. It may take years and the effects may be untraceable within the host of other factors now at play in our lives, but to microwave your food is to microwave yourself, and no other generation has ever tried that neat trick. It is best to cook on a gas stove, since it produces fire. Electrical elements are also a far cry from flame. Would you cook with fake water? Fake food? Better yet, move to Alaska and cook over open fires. Kidding. Sort of.

KEEP TV WATCHING TO A MINIMUM

I'm talking about one hour a day. TV is not just depressing; the vibrations it gives off are so yin that you feel totally depleted after too much TV, when you haven't really done anything. If you work at a computer, take frequent breaks and have lots of plants around you.

WALK IN NATURE

Take a walk outside for half an hour every day. You see, yin and yang are gunning for you, and their best shot comes when you get out in nature, away from the microwave, TV, and cell phone, bathing in the universe's vibes. Getting fresh air and moving your body in the great outdoors is very supportive to your overall health. When you can, take off your shoes and walk on dewy morning grass—a fantastic waker-upper and source of excellent-quality yin.

STAY ACTIVE

Get regular exercise. It doesn't much matter what you do, although as the food you eat gets milder in its intensity, your workouts may get a little milder. But don't worry—with less sludge in you, it takes less to move your vital life force around, which is all that exercise really is. So a light workout, a sweaty yoga class, or twenty minutes on the StairMaster may be all you need to stay fit.

BE GRATEFUL

Cultivate gratitude for life itself. With all the abundance you experience, it is only natural to give generously of your time and resources, so let the positive energy move through you, affecting the lives of others. This is perhaps the greatest high of all—impacting those we love in a positive way. As you eat whole grains, your soul sews up its wounds and it's easier to feel gratitude, as opposed to your emotional default mode being one of lack or self-pity. It also brings great perspective as you begin to look at life from an increasingly broader view. Investigate your ancestors. Trace the family tree. Begin to tune in to and appreciate the biological springboard from which you were launched.

TEACH OTHERS

But work with the ones who are genuinely interested; otherwise you'll end up feeling like an annoying, crazy hippy, which is unfortunate because you actually now have information that is extremely powerful and useful. Your own changes will be the greatest teachers to those around you, but don't be afraid to let people in on your macro secret.

HOME REMEDIES

I am only going to include a few home remedies, but you should know that there are many natural ways in which macrobiotic people treat their ills. From tofu compresses to sesame-ginger eyedrops to kombu tea, food can be used as medicine. Below are the ones I use most.

Ume-Sho-Kuzu

I love ume-sho-kuzu. Strengthening to the intestines, and therefore an overall power boost, this drink is an easy cure for diarrhea because the kuzu has a natural binding effect. It's also great after I have eaten sugar, because the umeboshi plum brings everything back to center, alkalizing the blood instantly. This is also a well-known remedy for hangovers, and if you have the presence of mind to make it be-

fore you go to bed, it's well worth it. This drink is good a couple of times a week for anyone with weak digestion. However, if you start to get constipated, skip the kuzu.

- 1 cup water
- ½ umeboshi plum
- 1 heaping teaspoon kuzu, diluted in ¼ cup cold spring water
- A few drops shoyu

Bring the water and ume plum to a boil. Simmer about 3 minutes. Add dilution of kuzu, stirring constantly to avoid lumps. Bring back to a boil. Add shoyu and let simmer about 4 more minutes. Drink/eat when it's come to a temperature you can handle, but the warmer the better.

Variation

Umeboshi tea (½ ume plum boiled in 1 cup water) is also good for hangovers, heartburn, and nausea.

Shiitake Mushroom Tea

Shiitake mushrooms are not only fat busters; they are also wonderful at pulling excess salt from the body. So after a salty Japanese meal, or when I just want to relax, I usually make myself some shiitake tea.

- 1 dried shiitake mushroom
- 1 cup of spring water
- 1–2 drops (literally) shoyu

Soak the mushroom in the water for 20 minutes. De-stem the soaked mushroom and slice the cap into strips. Bring water and mushroom to a boil. Simmer 10 minutes. Add shoyu and simmer 5 more. Drink.

Daikon Drink

This drink is great for relieving menstrual cramps and swollen ankles and feet. The smell created in your kitchen when the daikon is cooking might put you off, but it doesn't taste like the smell, and this drink's effects are well worth it.

- ½ cup grated (into a pulp) daikon
- ½ cup spring water
- 1–2 drops shoyu

Bring daikon and water to a boil. Add shoyu. Let simmer a couple of minutes. Drink/eat when temperature is right for you.

Carrot-Daikon Drink

This is a very common drink for people beginning a desludging diet. It has the power to really facilitate discharge, is a strong diuretic, and eliminates fats. But don't get addicted to this remedy. It is so powerful that, over time, it can be weakening. A couple of times a week should be enough unless your macrobiotic counselor says otherwise.

- ½ cup grated (into a pulp) carrot
- ½ cup grated (into a pulp) daikon
- ¼ umeboshi plum
- 1 cup spring water
- ¼ sheet nori, ripped into small pieces (optional)
- A few drops shoyu

Bring carrot, daikon, ume plum, and water to a boil. Let simmer about 3 minutes. Add nori if desired. Remove from heat and drink/eat.

CHAPTER EIGHT

more recipes

The following recipes are for generally healthy people who want to eat well, desludge, and find balance. Many of them are basic macrobiotic recipes that every good cook needs to master in order to manage his or her own health. So get well acquainted with these recipes, but be sure to read other macrobiotic cookbooks in order to expand your repertoire; I have only been able to cover a little territory of the vast expanse of macrobiotic cuisine.

grain products

Remember that *whole* grains are your leading men; these grain products, because they are cracked or pulverized into flour, have much less energy than whole grain. They are like Tony Soprano's thugs—necessary, but not the alpha male. Whole-grain recipes are on p. 83. The following dishes are delicious—so enjoy them but don't let them eclipse your whole grains.

Steamed Sourdough Bread

Bread can be addictive. Personally, I love sweets, but I have friends who would scramble right over my chocolate sundae for a nice, chewy baguette. The problem with bread is that it can leave the lover achy (especially in the neck and shoulders), irritable, and foggy brained. Sort of like a cute guy at the gym. Anyway, steamed bread—because it is not baked—is much softer, easier to digest, and an all-around gentler lover. It is also really easy to make. Steam yourself a loaf of sourdough every couple of weeks, eat it with onion butter or all-fruit jam, and you will never feel deprived.

- 2 level tablespoons miso
- 3 cups leftover rice or other grain
- 2½ cups whole-wheat bread flour
- ½ cup whole-wheat pastry flour
- Spring water
- Corn oil
- Raisins, seeds, onions, grated carrots, or other ingredients to add variety (optional)

Add miso to leftover rice, mixing them together well. Put aside for at least two days (I do three sometimes) in a warmish place. Massage it once a day to get the fermentation to occur. This will become a little smelly and wet. It is your sourdough "starter." The night before you plan to cook the bread, add the flour and water, a little at a time, until you are kneading a dense, but not inflexible, dough. Knead for a few minutes until the dough has a little springiness in it. *Note:* this dough will always be denser and less springy than white flour dough with conventional ingredients. Divide into two small loaves. Spread them lightly with corn oil. Cover with cheese-cloth and then a warm, damp towel. Let sit overnight. In the morning, place the dough (wrapped in cheesecloth) in a stainless-steel or bamboo steamer above a pot of boiling water. If you don't have a steamer, you might try putting it in a colander in a pot of boiling water, as long as the water doesn't come up to the level of the dough. Since the dough needs to steam for an hour, you must keep adding water to the pot. Check every 15 minutes or so to make sure you don't ruin your pot and your bread! Let cool and serve.

MAKES 12 SMALL SLICES OF BREAD

Fried Noodles

Dishes like fried noodles help me to stay macrobiotic. They are rich and soothing and can be made a myriad of ways, depending on your mood. If this recipe doesn't come out perfectly the first time—if the noodles stick, for example, or get a little soggy—fear not. Fried noodles is one of those dishes that you will develop your own personal "knack" for doing it your own way and intuiting the timing on things better and better over time. Practice this one at least once a week!

- 1 8-ounce package whole-wheat udon or soba noodles
- 2 tablespoons toasted sesame oil
- 1 onion, diced
- Pinch sea salt
- ½ carrot, cut into matchsticks
- 8 mushrooms, sliced
- 3 teaspoons shoyu
- Kernels from one ear corn
- 1 stalk bok choy, thinly sliced
- ¼ cup spring water
- 1 scallion, chopped
- Any other favorite vegetable that sautés well (optional)

Cook noodles according to instructions on package, drain, rinse with cold water, and set them aside. Heat oil in skillet and when hot (but not smoking) add onion. Add sea salt to bring out the onion's moisture and sweetness. Stir continually, as they become soft and translucent. Add carrots and continue to stir until they are slightly softened. Add mushrooms and sauté until moisture is released and they are soft. Season these vegetables with 1 teaspoon of the shoyu. Continue to stir as they cook another 2 minutes.

Add noodles on top. Do not stir them into the vegetables. Add corn and bok choy and the remaining 2 teaspoons of shoyu. Dribble in the spring water just to ensure that vegetables on bottom do not stick. Reduce heat to low and cover. Let it cook about 5 more minutes. The small amount of water produces enough steam to cook the dish but not enough to make the noodles soggy. Add scallion and toss. Serve hot.

MAKES 4 LARGE SERVINGS

Mochi Chips

Mochi is made from sweet brown rice steamed and pounded into a solid "cake." It is available at most health-food stores in a variety of flavors and is usually recooked in different ways.

- 1 package mochi
- Oil for deep-frying
- Shoyu or umeboshi vinegar (optional)
- Crumbled Kombu Chips (optional)

Slice mochi as thin as possible and let stand on a cookie sheet overnight. Fill 1-quart pot with 2 cups of oil. Heat oil to about 350°F. Test-fry one mochi chip by dropping it in. If the mochi drops to the bottom and then rises to the surface immediately—oil bubbling—the temperature is good for frying. If the mochi sinks to the bottom and rises slowly, it is not hot enough.

Deep-fry the mochi in batches so that the pot of oil does not become overcrowded or lose its heat. Remove from oil when the mochi crisps, puffs up, and rises to the top. Drain on paper towel. Spritz lightly with shoyu or umeboshi vinegar from a spray bottle if desired or sprinkle with crumbled Kombu Chips (see next recipe). Serve immediately.

SERVES 8

While you've got the hot oil going, try the following recipes:

Kombu Chips

This isn't a grain dish, but these kombu chips are tasty! So tasty, in fact, that you gotta go easy on them because they're a great way of getting a little too much salt. But, boy, oh boy, are they delicious.

- Two 2-inch strips dried kombu
- Safflower or sesame oil for frying

BEWARE: when the kombu is put in hot oil, it expands quickly and spits lots of oil. So be careful and either have a splatter screen to put on top of the oil or step away quicky. The kombu cooks very fast and should be taken out almost as soon as it's put in.

With oil at 350°F, place strips of kombu in oil until they expand and bubble a little. With a slotted spoon or skimmer, take out kombu and place on paper towel to dry.

SERVES 1

Mochi Waffles

For this, you need a waffle iron, which runs from about thirty to fifty bucks in any department store and—if it's good quality—will serve you well.

- 1 package mochi, plain or flavored

Recommended Toppings
- All-fruit jam
- Nut butters
- Rice syrup
- Maple syrup
- Tahini-miso spread
- Squash or onion butter
- Tahini with raspberry-flavored rice syrup (my favorite)
- Cooked fruit
- Dried fruit compote

Grate the mochi or cut it into thin slices, about ⅛-inch thick. When the waffle iron is ready, place a small handful of the mochi in the waffle iron. Close the top and apply a little pressure. You can either continue to apply pressure or just wait. The waffle iron (if electric) should have a light that goes either on or off to indicate that the waffle is ready. Remove light, airy waffle from iron and slather with your favorite topping.

SERVES 4

Hambulghur Helper

Quick, light, and easy, this dish only needs some steamed or boiled greens to make it into a satisfying meal.

- Toasted sesame oil to fry tempeh, plus 1 tablespoon
- 8 ounces tempeh, sliced into bite-sized cubes
- 1 medium onion, diced
- ⅛ teaspoon sea salt
- 1 large carrot, cut into matchsticks

- 2 cups bulghur wheat
- 1 cup whole-wheat rotini or elbow noodles
- 5 cups spring water
- 3 tablespoons shoyu
- 2 tablespoons mirin
- ⅛ teaspoon brown rice vinegar
- Kernels from 1 ear corn
- 2 stalks celery, diced

In a large frying pan, heat sesame oil over medium heat. When hot (but not smoking,) add tempeh, frying the cubes until browned and crispy. Remove from heat and let drain on paper towel. Set aside.

In a large saucepan, heat 1 tablespoon of sesame oil over medium heat. Add onion and salt and sauté until translucent. Add carrot and sauté for a few minutes. Pour in bulghur wheat and noodles, stirring them into the vegetables. Fold in tempeh. Mix water, shoyu, mirin, and vinegar altogether, and add to pot. Bring to a boil uncovered, reduce flame to low, cover, and place on flame deflector. Let simmer 15 minutes. Add corn and celery. Cook for 5 more minutes. Remove from heat and let sit a couple of minutes to prevent sticking. Serve.

SERVES 8

vegetables

I'm not going to waste my time telling you that vegetables are good for you. Your mother's voice echoing, "Eat your vegetables—they're good for you," should have done the trick. What's fascinating about vegetables is that not only are they amazing for you, but they each deliver a different energy or essense to different parts of the body. In macrobiotics, we basically break vegetables into three categories: upward, round (or ground), and downward.

UPWARD-GROWING VEGETABLES

These guys are so great! They include kale, collard greens, watercress, leeks, mustard greens, Chinese cabbage (nappa), carrot tops, daikon tops, turnip tops, parsley, scallions, mizuma, celery, sprouts, chives, lettuce, and endive.

Greens are *full* of minerals, so they are strenghthening and good for your blood, which needs chlorophyll and stuff like calcium and iron. The energy they impart is upward and is especially friendly to the liver, lungs, and brain. If you are feeling sludgy or less than perky, eat a serving of blanched leafy greens in the morning and you will brighten up immediately. I eat some kind of upward-growing vegetable at every meal. They are cooling and relaxing in a good-quality, clearheaded way. But if you eat *only* leafy greens, you will get sort of scattered and ungrounded. Keep in mind that spinach and chard, both high in oxalic acid, are generally not used.

ROUND OR GROUND VEGETABLES

They include squash (acorn, butternut, buttercup, Hubbard, pumpkin, hokkaido pumpkin—also summer squash and pattypan), rutabaga, turnip, brussels sprouts, onion, green cabbage, red cabbage, cauliflower, cucumber, green peas, green beans, mushrooms, and Jerusalem artichokes. These vegetables, especially the round, sweet ones, have a soothing and centering effect on the body. They appeal to and relax the middle organs—stomach, liver, spleen, and pancreas. Cooking styles like nishime also deliver mellow, warming energy to the body. Potatoes, tomatoes, and eggplant—members of the nightshade family and considered dangerously yin—are generally avoided.

DOWNWARD-GROWING VEGETABLES

This category includes carrot, burdock, parsnip, daikon, radish, lotus root, and dandelion root. The intestines are the "roots" of our digestion and, therefore, our overall health. Root-vegetable energy is grounding and helps digestive function. These vegetables help to keep energy centered and inward. Lotus root has the particular quality of pulling excess fluid from the lungs and large intestine.

JUGGLING VEGETABLES

I was agog when I found out that it wasn't right for me to break down the vegetable categories into perfect thirds. Because yang energy is so strong, similar volumes of yin and yang foods are not necessarily equal, just as a cup of salt and a cup of sugar do not balance each other. Most people need more greens to feel balanced and happy. Try one-half green and upward, one-quarter round, and one-quarter down. Or two-thirds and one-sixth and one-sixth. Of course, this doesn't have to be measured, just eyeballed. See what feels right to you.

COOKING STYLES

Each cooking style completely changes the character of a food. Carrot soup is a very different thing than grated carrot in a salad. As you play with vegetables, understand that they are fascinating and wily characters: a pungent turnip becomes sweet when cooked; red onions roasted with olive oil, salt, and rosemary are distant cousins to those cooked in a nishime. As much as the vegetable imparts a certain energy, the way it is prepared has an equal impact. By using time, heat, pressure, salt, water, and oil, we change the character and direction the vegetable's energy takes in the body. Try all the following cooking styes and experiment madly within the amazing world of vegetables.

long-cooked vegetable dishes

In general, cooking something slowly and over a long time has a warming and energizing effect on the body. When animal food is not depended upon for internal heat and energy, strong cooking styles deliver the punch. So, far from being a no-no, deep-frying is an important cooking style because it brings quick and active heat to the body. Nishime, kimpira, and long sautés bring warmth and groundedness to the middle organs and intestines. As you eat more whole foods, your intuition will awaken to exactly what you need and the cooking style that brings it.

Nishime Vegetables

Also known as "waterless cooking," nishime-style cooking involves hearty, sweet vegetables steamed slowly in their own juices. What results is a potful of chunky, delicious, fall-apart vegetables that go down like butter. This dish has a centering effect on the body and mind and is unbelievably simple given the level of satisfaction it produces. If you are feeling scattered and out of sorts, use a nishime to come home to yourself. Make nishime vegetables at least a couple of times a week, using different vegetables depending on the season.

- 1-inch piece dried kombu
- 1 medium onion, cut into thick wedges
- 6 inches daikon, cut into thick rounds
- 3 medium parsnips, cut into thick diagonal slices
- 2 medium carrots, cut into 2-inch "logs"
- Spring water
- ½ teaspoon shoyu

In a heavy pot with a heavy lid (preferably enameled cast iron) place the dried kombu. Add the onion. Layer the daikon, carrots, and parsnips, respectively. Pour roughly 1 inch of spring water into the pot. Cover and bring to a boil. Reduce heat and let simmer 10–15 minutes or until carrots are soft. Season with shoyu and simmer 5 more minutes. Remove the kombu and discard or slice into thin strips and return to pot. Serve.

SERVES 8

Variation

A summer-style nishime might include carrots, summer squash, and green beans.

Rutabaga Fries

- 1 large rutabaga
- 2–3 tablespoons extra-virgin olive oil
- ½ teaspoon sea salt

Preheat oven to 400°F. Wash rutabaga and cut into french-fry-sized sticks. Place in bowl and mix in olive oil and salt until the sticks are well coated. Roast on a baking sheet until brown and crispy—about 40 minutes.

SERVES 4

Variation

Roasted vegetables in general are a great thing. Try red onion, mushrooms, summer squash, carrots, and lightly blanched broccoli with olive oil, salt, and some dried rosemary. Reduce cooking time to 15–20 minutes for these lighter vegetables.

Onion Butter

I used to cook professionally with my then-boyfriend, Howard. One night we were making onion butter for a family we were working for, and after sautéing the sliced onions, we let them cook a little and then completely forgot about them. In the middle of the night, Howard woke up like someone seeing a ghost, half whispering, half shrieking, "The onions! The onions!" Instead of waking up the whole house, we just crossed our fingers and went back to sleep. In the morning, we served up the most delicious, rich, sweet, caramelized onion butter ever made, acting as if it turned out that well all the time.

- 6 medium onions, sliced into thin half-moons
- 3 tablespoons untoasted sesame or olive oil
- 1 teaspoon sea salt
- Spring water (if needed)

Heat the oil in a cast-iron or enameled cast-iron pot. Make sure whatever you use has a heavy lid. Add onions when oil is hot and sprinkle the salt in to draw out the onions' sweetness and moisture. Sauté until onions are translucent. Considering the amount of onions, this may take a little while. Add a tiny bit of water if it seems dry or if the onions are sticking to the bottom of the pot. Cover and reduce heat to very low, putting a flame deflector under the pot. The heavy lid of the pot will keep all the cooking juices in, and the onions should not burn. Simmer for anywhere between 3 hours and overnight until onions are completely reduced and really sweet. Make sure if you leave it overnight that the pot is on two flame deflectors over a low flame. Serve as a snack, on sourdough bread or rice cakes.

THIS RECIPE MAKES 6 SERVINGS
*(at 3 hours of cooking), although the longer the onions cook,
the sweeter and more reduced they become.*

Purple Passion Stew

Technically not a stew, this dish is a variation on nishime-style cooking. Its bright purple color and slighty sour taste make for a bold, exotic character on the plate. This particular hue, almost a fuschia, is a great complement to the bright greens and oranges of other vegetables.

- 2-inch piece kombu, soaked and sliced into thin strips
- 1 medium daikon, sliced into 1-inch rounds
- ½ small red cabbage *or* ¼ large red cabbage, chopped into bite-sized chunks
- Spring water
- 1 tablespoon umeboshi vinegar

Place the soaked kombu slices in the bottom of a heavy pot. Add daikon rounds and then place cabbage on top. Pour about 1 inch of water into the pot. Add umeboshi vinegar. Cover and bring to a boil. Reduce flame to low and simmer for 30 minutes. Remove from heat and stir so that the daikon gets stained purple.

SERVES 4

Tempura

And you thought you had to go out and pay lots of money to eat tempura! Not anymore. Tempura is incredibly cheap, easy, and fun to make. And don't get weirded out about deep-frying, because tempura that's done correctly doesn't have that much oil in it. At the same time, tempura gives very strong, hot, active energy to the body while delivering quality ingredients.

Batter
- 1 cup whole-wheat pastry flour
- ¼ teaspoon sea salt
- 2 level teaspoons kuzu, diluted in a little cold spring water
- 1–1¼ cups spring water

- Sesame or safflower oil for frying

To Be Tempuraed
- Carrots, cut on a medium-thick diagonal

- Broccoli florets
- Cauliflower florets
- Green beans
- Mushrooms
- Brussels sprouts
- Squash or sweet potato
- Celery
- Onions
- Burdock
- Tofu
- Seitan
- Nori seaweed*
- Parsley*
- Kale
- Apple
- Anything you want to try

Prep vegetables by washing, cutting, and drying them carefully. Tempura works best if the vegetables are dry. Mix dry ingredients of batter and add kuzu and water. Stir well to get rid of lumps. The batter will thicken a little in a few minutes. (It may seem thin, but try deep-frying a vegetable before adding more flour.)

Bring 2–3 inches of oil to 350°F in a small or medium-sized pot over medium heat. You can test the oil by dropping a small amount of tempura batter in it. If it sinks and then rises to the surface quickly, bubbling strongly, it is ready. Avoid letting the oil get so hot that it smokes. Deep-fry a few vegetables at a time, allowing them to cook until the batter looks slightly golden. Then turn them over and let the other side become the same color. Remove with wire mesh strainer. Drain on paper towel. If you are doing a big batch, let the finished tempura warm on a cookie sheet in a 200°F oven. When you're done with the oil, strain it for debris; then, while it's still hot, deep-fry an umeboshi pit until it is

---

*Make sure you try. Tempuraed nori tastes like a great deep-fried fish dish.

charred. This will get rid of any odors. Deep-fry oil can be reused two more times.

MAKES 12 PIECES, WHICH WILL SERVE 3 PEOPLE

Dip Sauces

These dip sauces give tempura eating the strong dynamic energy we all love. Guests should get a little bowl of their own dip sauce. Lots of tempura dip sauces include daikon, which helps to digest the oil, but if you choose a dip sauce without it, grate a little daikon and serve it on the side.

Dip Sauce #1
- ¼ teaspoon grated daikon
- 1 tablespoon shoyu
- 2 tablespoons spring water

Dip Sauce #2
- ⅛ teaspoon grated ginger
- 1 tablespoon shoyu
- 2 tablespoons spring water

EACH SAUCE SERVES 1

Kinpira

Kinpira is a traditional Japanese dish for giving energy and strengthening the intestines. Burdock, an incredibly tough, yang root vegetable, is a blood strengthener and purifier. If you want to get something accomplished, and you've been dillydallying, cook and eat a serving of kinpira. The job will get done. Try this recipe a couple of times a week.

- 1–2 tablespoons toasted sesame oil
- 1 medium burdock root, cut into fine matchsticks
- 2 medium carrots, cut into fine matchsticks
- 1 pinch sea salt
- 2 tablespoons spring water
- shoyu*
- ginger juice

Heat the oil in a heavy skillet that has a lid. Sauté burdock first, stirring constantly for about 3 minutes. Add the carrots and salt, stirring for another 3 minutes. Sprinkle the water over the vegetables, cover, and reduce to low, allowing vegetables to steam. After 10–15 minutes, open and check to see that the dish is relatively dry. Add a sprinkle of shoyu. Cover and cook 5 more minutes. Add a few drops of ginger juice. Serve while hot.

SERVES 6

---

*Kinpira is a traditionally strengthening dish (yang), so it's not unusual for it to be well seasoned. Add more shoyu if the dish feels underseasoned, but go light on the shoyu if you are feeling too yang (see pages 271–273).

Dried Daikon with Dried Tofu

Daikon is the greatest food. Fresh grated daikon has the power to cut totally through oil and fat served in a meal; that's why it always accompanies tempura in Japanese restaurants. Dried daikon has the power to dissolve fats found deeper in the body—the really old sludge. For maximum sludge-busting, make a dried daikon dish every week! Keep in mind that everything is always changing, and dried daikon gets old; look for daikon that is still a beautiful, yellowish gold color. If it's brown, it's getting old and bitter.

- ½ package dried daikon (about 1 cup)
- 2 squares dried tofu (optional)

- Spring water for soaking
- 1 cup spring water
- 3 tablespoons shoyu
- 1 tablespoon extra-virgin olive oil or toasted sesame oil
- 1 medium onion, sliced into half-moons
- Pinch sea salt
- 1 medium carrot, cut into matchsticks
- Chopped scallions for garnish

Soak the daikon in water for 30 minutes. If the soaking water turns a light gold color and tastes sweet, you can use it in the dish. If it turns brown or tastes bitter, discard it and cook with fresh water. If using dried tofu, soak it for 5 minutes in spring water and then squeeze out all the liquid. Then marinate tofu in water with 2 tablespoons of the shoyu until needed. Heat oil in heavy skillet and sauté onion with the salt until onion is translucent. Add carrot and sauté a few more minutes. Squeeze excess liquid out of dried daikon and cut into 1-inch pieces. If also using tofu, squeeze the excess marinade from it and slice the tofu into ½-inch strips.

Place the daikon onto the vegetables and (if using) the tofu on the daikon. Add daikon soaking water (or fresh water) to the skillet, going roughly halfway up the daikon/vegetable mixture. Cover and bring to a boil. Reduce heat and simmer 25 minutes. Check occasionally in case small amounts of liquid are needed. But don't go overboard—this dish should not come out watery. Add the remaining shoyu and cook 5 more minutes. Garnish and serve.

SERVES 4

Variation

Try doing this same recipe with dried shiitake mushrooms and sliced kombu. Or try snow peas, fresh corn, or fresh green beans cooked in at the end to lighten it up.

lightly cooked vegetable dishes

Steamed Greens

Greens, rich in chlorophyll and minerals like calcium, strengthen the bones, help the blood to absorb oxygen, and bring energy upward in the body, leaving you feeling light and refreshed. Because greens have absorbed so much light, they are like "eating sunshine."

- 1 bunch collard greens or kale
- Spring water for boiling

Wash the greens thoroughly and separate the green leaf from the tough stem by slicing carefully along each side of the stem. Cut the stem into tiny rounds. Slice the greens into 1-inch strips. Bring water to a boil and steam the greens (and stem bits) in a steamer on top or place them in a steaming basket within the pot. Cover and let steam for 3–5 minutes. The greens will go from their raw color to a very brilliant green, then a deeper green and, if overcooked, look dull. If you really overcook them, they'll appear a little brownish.

After 3 minutes, first check the color and then taste one piece—they are best at their deep green color. If they are tough or unchewably fibrous, let them cook another minute or so. As your intuition becomes sharper and sharper, you will cook greens well consistently. Over time, you will find that you simply "know" when they're ready.

MAKES 4–6 SERVINGS
depending on the size of the greens

Sautéed Vegetables

Sautéed vegetables keep me alive during the summer. They are quick and delicious, and the energy is perfect for warm weather. But because of the oil, sautéed vegetables are also totally appropriate for colder months. Health food never tasted so good.

- 1–2 tablespoons sesame or olive oil
- 1 clove garlic, minced
- Pinch sea salt
- 12 mushrooms, sliced
- 1 cup snow peas
- Kernels from 1 ear corn
- 2 stalks bok choy, cut into 1-inch pieces
- ½ teaspoon shoyu
- 3 tablespoons spring water

Heat oil over medium heat in skillet or wok. Add garlic and salt, stirring constantly for about 10 seconds. Add mushrooms and stir until they begin to soften. Add snow peas, corn, bok choy, and shoyu. Stir to get everything together. Add the spring water and cover. This small amount of water will steam the vegetables. Cook for 4 minutes. Remove from heat and serve immediately.

SERVES 4

Variations

Red onion, carrots, boy choy, and nori seaweed, seasoned with shoyu. Burdock, collard greens, umeboshi vinegar, and ginger juice.

Tip

With any combination of vegetables, simply start with the heartiest vegetable and end with the softest.

Boiled Salad with Pumpkin-Seed Dressing

I know, I know. It sounds as though someone just dunked a raw salad in boiling water, and that's not terribly appetizing. This dish is actually a "salad" of lightly blanched vegetables. I didn't really like boiled salads until I learned this version from Denny Waxman, a macrobiotic counselor in Philadelphia. Check out his Web site at strengtheninghealth.org. Now I like boiled salads so much, I arrange the vegetables in colorful patterns and structures that are so strange that a rich, famous artiste client we once cooked for always looked forward to my next boiled salad. I was flattered.* So be creative, play with quantities, and mix and match with a variety of colorful vegetables. Boil salads—big and small—will keep you fresh, light, and perky.

- Red onion
- Green cabbage
- Red cabbage
- Radishes
- Daikon
- Carrots
- Leeks
- Kale
- Bok choy
- Green beans
- Snow peas
- Collard greens
- Nappa cabbage
- Squash
- Summer squash

---

*It is not necessary, or even desirable, to make a dressing for every boiled salad. If you feel that you are getting too much salt, or identify with the symptoms of becoming too yang (see p. 255), skip the dressing or lighten the seasoning within it significantly. A fresh, plain boiled salad tastes great on its own.

- Mustard greens
- Any other vegetable that strikes your fancy

- 1 grain sea salt

Wash and slice vegetables in thin slices. Bring a pot of water to a boil. Add sea salt—no more than the 1 grain, if possible. Even one grain of sea salt draws the minerals and taste to the periphery of the vegetable. Take one type of vegetable and place in the water. Immediately *turn off heat*. Just let the vegetable sit in the water for about a minute (hearty greens may need longer). Because the water is no longer actively boiling, the minerals and flavor stay in the vegetable instead of being released into the water. This is what makes them so delicious. Remove with slotted spoon and put aside. You can, if you wish, run cold water over the vegetable to maintain a bright color. Bring the water to a boil again (no need to add more salt) and cook the next vegetable. Turn off heat and repeat as above. When all the vegetables are done, arrange them in an attractive way on a platter. Serve as is or with Pumpkin-Seed Dressing (see next recipe).

Tip

Cook any vegetables with a bitter taste, like mustard greens and radishes, at the end, since they make the cooking water kind of bitter.

Pumpkin-Seed Dressing

This dressing is as delicious as it is simple. Great for boiled salads, pressed salads, or as a dip, it keeps in the fridge for about a week.

- 1 cup unroasted pumpkin seeds
- Pulp of 2 umeboshi plums *or* 1½ tablespoons umeboshi paste *or* 1½ tablespoons umeboshi vinegar
- 1–2 cups spring water

Rinse the pumpkin seeds and get rid of any broken or weird-looking seeds. Heat a cast-iron or stainless-steel skillet over medium heat. Add seeds and move them briskly with a wooden spoon over heat until they are dry. Reduce heat to low and continue to agitate the seeds either with a spoon or by sautéing them. The seeds should puff up or pop. When most of them have expanded, remove from heat. Let the seeds cool a little. Then pour them into a blender or food processor. Blend the dry seeds until they are a grainy powder. Add the flesh of the umeboshi plums and about half of the water. Blend and continue to slowly add the remainder of the water until smooth. Continue to add umeboshi or water until you reach the consistency and taste of a dressing that you desire.

MAKES 2 CUPS

Variation

If you have extra time, grind the seeds in suribachi. Add seasoning and water, grinding until dressing is the desired consistency.

Teaser Caesar

This version of a Caesar salad was something that Howard and I came upon in Vegetarian Times *magazine. The nutritional yeast is the only ingredient that may not work for people going whole hog, but it's so good, I just had to include it.*

Croutons
- 3–4 slices whole-wheat sourdough bread, sliced into cubes (about 1½ cups)
- Olive oil
- ½ teaspoon dried rosemary
- ½ teaspoon dried marjoram
- ½ teaspoon garlic powder
- ½ teaspoon sea salt

Preheat over to 325°F. Lightly coat bread slices with olive oil. In a small bowl, mix remaining crouton ingredients. Add bread; toss to coat. Spread in a single layer on baking sheet. Bake until croutons are dry and lightly toasted, 10–5 minutes. Remove from oven and set aside.

Dressing

- 2 tablespoons blanched or roasted almonds
- 3 cloves garlic, minced
- 3 tablespoons Dijon mustard
- 1 tablespoon nutritional yeast flakes*
- 2 tablespoons shoyu
- 1 tablespoon tahini
- 3 tablespoons fresh lemon juice
- ¼ cup water
- 2 tablespoons extra-virgin olive oil
- 1 large head romaine lettuce, torn into large pieces

Meanwhile, in food processor or blender, combine almonds, garlic, mustard, yeast flakes, shoyu, tahini, lemon juice, water, and oil; process until smooth and well blended. To serve, toss together lettuce and croutons. Add dressing and toss to coat. Serve right away.

SERVES 6–8

---

*Nutritional yeast is not normally used in macrobiotic cooking. If you're following a clean, whole-hog regime, skip it.

Colorful Harvest Salad
(A Pressed Salad)

This recipe is by Jane Quincannon, a wonderful southern belle, a good friend, and a longtime macrobiotica. This colorful, crisp, and satisfying salad brightens any table, any season. Pressing gives the salad greater digestibility and tenderness and blends the flavors to create a delicious, refreshing, healthful vegetable dish that is packed with minerals, phyto-nutrients, and beta-carotene.

- ⅓ cup thinly sliced red cabbage
- ½ cup thinly sliced Nappa cabbage
- ½ cup carrot, cut into thin matchsticks
- ½ teaspoon sea salt
- ½ cup thinly sliced Granny Smith apple
- 2 drops umeboshi and/or brown rice vinegar, or to taste (optional)
- 1 shake dulse flakes
- 2 tablespoons chopped roasted walnuts (optional)

Slice vegetables as thinly as possible. Mix all together in a large mixing bowl. Add sea salt, mix, and gently squeeze with your hands. A small amount of water should begin to drip from the vegetables. Gently mix in the apples and place the salad into a salad press or into a bowl with a plate to cover the vegetables; then place a jar or small weight on top of the plate. Press the salad for 30 minutes or longer until water is expelled out of the vegetables. Discard water and rinse salad in a strainer twice. Squeeze out water from the salad and place in bowl. If desired, you may season the salad with umeboshi and/or brown rice vinegar. Mix in the dulse flakes and, if desired, the walnuts.

SERVES 4

Variation

Add minced dark greens such as watercress, parsley, dandelion, etc.

Mock Greek Salad
(A Pressed Salad)

As you've probably noticed, I lean on my friends because I am not a natural-born artist in the kitchen. However, this is one of my original recipes, what I thunk up myself.

- 4 ounces firm tofu
- 2 tablespoons umeboshi vinegar
- 4 cups (chopped into ½–1-inch pieces) Nappa cabbage
- ½ medium cucumber, sliced into ¼-inch-thick half-moons
- ¼ red onion, sliced into thin half-moons
- 8 Kalamata olives, sliced lengthwise into quarters

Crumble tofu and mix with 1 tablespoon of the vinegar. Set aside. Add the other tablespoon of ume vinegar to the Napa cabbage, cucumbers, and red onion in a large bowl or pickle press. Massage them all together with your hands until the vegetables begin to "sweat." Press the mixture in a pickle press or create pressure by placing a plate on the vegetables and a heavy weight on the plate. Press for 20 minutes (or, for a lighter dish, don't press at all). Pour off excess liquid (rinse if too salty for your taste). Add olives and crumbled tofu. Serve.

SERVES 4–6

Nabe (Na-Bay)-Style
Vegetables

When I was living in a macro community and I was getting way too yang, everyone kept saying, "Make nabe, make nabe!" which drove me completely crazy because I was too yang and therefore everything drove me crazy. Anyway, I finally surrendered, and one night in my apartment I made myself a mess of nabe-style vegetables. The next morning, I felt so light and happy, I couldn't believe it. I know it sounds crazy, but this stuff is true. The secret is in the kombu and the shiitake and how they interact with the vegetables.

This recipe is really lovely and different done in a ceramic pot (nabe means "pot," and ceramic pots for this dish are sold in some health-food stores—not expensive) but is fine in stainless steel as well. It is often cooked at the table over a single gas burner so that the family can all dig in at once.

IMPORTANT: nabe meals are meant to be relaxing, uplifting affairs, so about two-thirds of the vegetables done are upward and green, while only one-third are downward and hearty. Also less grain should be served at the meal than at a normal meal. Nabe-centered meals include less grain than other meals. The following recipe yields no particular amount because it is up to you to decide how much you want or need to eat.

- 1 2-inch piece kombu
- 2 dried shiitake mushrooms
- Spring water

Stuff for the Nabe
- Carrots
- Onions
- Broccoli
- Cauliflower
- Burdock
- Mushrooms
- Kale
- Collards
- Nappa cabbage
- Green cabbage
- Bok choy
- Leeks
- Mustard greens
- Radishes and their tops
- Daikon
- Lotus root

- Any other vegetable you want
- Tofu
- Mochi
- Seitan

Soak kombu and shiitake mushrooms in water that goes halfway up a 4-quart (or larger) saucepan for 5–10 minutes. When they are soft, slice them into thin strips and return to water. Place the saucepan over medium-high heat and bring water to a boil. Meanwhile, prepare vegetables by cleaning them and cutting into bite-sized pieces. Carrots and burdock are best cut on a diagonal. Slice mushrooms and radishes in half. Onions are best in thick wedges.

When the water comes to a boil, place a few groups of vegetables in the water. Each type of vegetable is ready at a different time, and it is not important that you catch the vegetable at its peak. When nabe is cooked over a portable gas cooker in the middle of the family table, some vegetables stay in the pot a very long time.

When some vegetables look ready, lift them out with a slotted spoon and replace them with raw ones. Just keep removing and replacing, either eating as you go or doing it until you have a nice variety of vegetables to serve. The whole process could take 15–20 minutes.

Nabe Dip Sauce

It is not necessary to have a dip sauce every time you make nabe, since it can be a way of getting too much salt over time. If you're feeling pressured or irritable, skip the dip. It is customary for each person to have their own bowl of dip sauce.

- 1 cup water left over from nabe cooking (or spring water)
- 2 tablespoons shoyu
- 1 tablespoon minced scallions for garnish
- 1 teaspoon grated ginger

If using nabe water, after the last vegetable is done, just season the broth, simmer 4 minutes, and garnish with scallions. Squeeze the grated ginger over the bowl until a few drops of juice drip into the sauce. If using plain water, just bring it to a boil, add seasoning, and simmer 4 minutes. Garnish with scallions and ginger juice. For a stronger dip sauce, add more ginger and shoyu.

SERVES 2

Roots and Tops

This is great dish because it's quick and refreshing and totally packs a punch. By keeping the roots and the tops together, we're bringing back Starsky and Hutch, Mick and Keith, Laurel and Hardy—individuals who aren't half as powerful on their own. But together, they are magic.

- 2 carrots *or* 2 parsnips *or* 1 daikon, sliced on a thin diagonal; *or* 4 red radishes, halved or quartered
- Spring water
- The corresponding leafy top of the vegetable, cleaned and sliced into 1-inch pieces
- ½ teaspoon shoyu
- 2 teaspoons toasted sesame seeds

Place sliced root in a pot with water to almost cover. Bring to a boil covered, and let simmer about 1 minute. Add the tops and shoyu, cover, and let simmer 3 more minutes. Remove from heat. Toss with sesame seeds and serve hot. *Yum.*

SERVES 2-4

beans

You're probably familiar with beans. Either you eat them regularly already or you avoid them like the plague because they give you gas. Beans are really great foods, for lots of reasons, but their fartiness gives them a bad rap. Let's address that first:

Beans make you toot: but they don't have to. Soaking and cooking beans with kombu reduce their gassiness, as does removing any foam that occurs in the cooking process. However, the best defense against gas is chewing beans really well. You should be an excellent chewer by now, but if you haven't practiced much, try with beans. Chew beans fifty to a hundred times a mouthful. The digestive enzymes in your mouth set up all the other digestive enzymes in your body and make beans a much, much friendlier experience.

Beans are high in protein: although they contain all eight essential amino acids that make up protein, beans have a special relationship with grains, and together the two create a protein that is very easily assimilated. But it's also good to understand that our society's virtual paranoia about not getting enough protein is unfounded. The truth is, most of our diseases are those of excess; it is actually very difficult to become protein deficient, and it can be argued that we get way too much protein. Beans are a very respectable, healthy source of protein. Eat them within a diet of whole grains, vegetables, and other healthy foods, and you'll be fine.

Beans have healing properties: meat gives strong energy but doesn't have any particularly healing properties—in fact, quite the opposite. Beans are considered especially nourishing to the kidneys, but each type of bean has its distinct healing qualities. In order to receive this magic all over, it is important that you eat a broad variety of beans.

Beans are rich, dense, and heavy: they are downright yummy and satisfying. That's a very important quality in feeling nourished and grounded. Too many beans can make you feel sluggish, but you will find what's right for you.

Red Lentil–Walnut Pâté

This is an adaptation of another amazing Christina Pirello recipe that she has given me permission to use. I confided in her that I liked to "up the volume" on the seasonings in this recipe, and she gave me an enthusiastic "Go for it!"

- 2 cups dried red lentils, sorted and rinsed well
- 1 2-inch piece wakame, soaked and diced
- 4 cups spring water
- 1 tablespoon shoyu
- 1 tablespoon extra-virgin olive oil
- 1 onion, diced
- 3 cloves garlic, minced
- ½ teaspoon dried basil
- 1½ cups lightly pan-toasted walnut pieces
- ¼ cup minced fresh parsley
- 2 tablespoons umeboshi vinegar
- 2 tablespoons balsamic vinegar

Place lentils, wakame, and water in a heavy pot over medium heat. Bring to a boil and boil, uncovered, 10 minutes. Reduce heat, cover, and simmer 20 minutes (or until lentils are creamy, which could be much sooner). Season lightly with shoyu and simmer 5 minutes.

Meanwhile, heat oil in a skillet over medium heat. Add onion, garlic, and basil and cook, stirring, 3–4 minutes or until softened. Set aside.

Transfer cooked beans, vegetables, walnuts, parsley, and vinegars to a food processor. Puree until smooth and creamy. Serve with raw or lightly blanched vegetables, rice crackers, or toasted pita bread.

SERVES 8

Aduki Beans with Squash and Kombu

This is a simple, medicinal recipe. Aduki beans, native to Japan but also now cultivated in the United States, are small burgundy-colored beans that are very nurturing to the kidneys. In Oriental medicine, the strength of the kidneys is an indicator of overall strength. Weak, depleted kidneys and overworked adrenal glands are the by-products of too much sugar, alcohol, caffeine, and stress. The sweet squash in this recipe serves as a tonic to the stomach, spleen, and pancreas, helping to keep blood sugar even and stabilize your mood. Kombu, the sea vegetable used to help soften the beans, thus making them more digestible, is also rich in lovely minerals.

- A 4–6-inch piece kombu
- 1 cup aduki beans
- Spring water
- 2 cups hard winter squash, cut into chunks and unpeeled if organic
- 1 teaspoon shoyu

Combine the kombu and the beans and soak overnight. After soaking, remove the kombu from the beans and discard the soaking water. Slice the reconstituted kombu into 1-inch-by-1-inch squares and place them in the bottom of a heavy pot with a heavy lid, preferably enameled cast iron. Add the beans on top of the kombu. Add fresh spring water to just cover the beans. Bring to a boil uncovered. When it boils, strain off any foam that might be floating on top. Let the beans boil for about 5 minutes uncovered, as this allows gases to release into the air, and not through you later on. Cover the pot, place a flame deflector beneath it, and reduce heat to a simmer. Let the beans cook for about 40 minutes, adding water when it appears to dip down below the bean level. Check them every 10 minutes or so. Add the squash on top of the beans and add more water— to cover the beans—if necessary. Let this cook for another 20 minutes. When the beans seem soft and tender, add the shoyu and let them cook 10 more minutes. Stir a little to mix the beans and squash and serve.

SERVES 6

Variation

Add the squash from the beginning of the simmering of the beans. This will make the squash melt more into the beans, creating a softer dish. Try it both ways and see what you like.

Mock Tuna

No, you're not making fun of a fish. This recipe is for those of us who had a very intimate relationship with little cans in our cupboards and who miss the idea of opening them regularly. Tuna is very yang and contracting—considered too strong an energy to take in regularly, especially for a woman. Ditto salmon. Macrobiotic recipes generally stick to white-fleshed fish that are lower in fat and more easily digestible. Therefore, to imitate the sensual pleasure of tuna fish, we use tempeh.

- 1 8-ounce package tempeh
- 1 tablespoon umeboshi vinegar
- ⅓ cup Tofu Mayonnaise (see p. 123 or store-bought)
- Black pepper to taste
- Any spices you desire—cumin, curry, paprika, saffron, etc. (optional)
- 1 celery stalk, diced
- ¼ red onion, finely diced

Steam or boil tempeh for 20 minutes to make it more digestible. Break apart with a fork until you get smaller-than-bite-sized pieces. Sprinkle the umeboshi vinegar onto the tempeh, mashing it in with a fork until you get a tuna-fishy saltiness. Mix "mayonnaise," pepper, and any other spices you enjoy. Mash into tempeh. Add vegetables. Serve or refrigerate—it tastes even better the next day.

SERVES 4

Hummus

Hummus is a very personal thing. When I cooked with Howard, he insisted on making the hummus because he felt his ethnic heritage gave him special insight into the matter that my Scottish roots did not. But I watched him, and I learned a thing or two. Like hummus is never the same thing twice. Start with this recipe, but experiment madly. Are you someone who likes to taste the olive oil? Likes more garlic? Lemon? Be bold.

- 1 cup chickpeas, soaked overnight with 2-inch piece kombu *or* 2 cans precooked chickpeas
- Spring water
- ½ teaspoon sea salt
- 2 tablespoons umeboshi paste
- 2 tablespoons olive oil
- 1 clove garlic, minced
- 1 tablespoon tahini
- 2 tablespoons lemon juice

If you are cooking the chickpeas: discard soaking water. Slice kombu into strips and place on the bottom of a pressure cooker. Add chickpeas. Add water to just cover the beans. Let them come to a boil uncovered. Skim off any foam that might arise. Close the pressure cooker and bring to full pressure, then place flame deflector under it and reduce heat to low. Let cook 1¼ hours. Remove from heat, allow pressure to come down, open the pot, and add salt. Let cook 10 more minutes.

In a food processor, blend chickpeas and the rest of the ingredients. Serve with steamed sourdough pita bread, rice cakes, or raw vegetables.

SERVES 6

Variation

My mother puts about 1 tablespoon of fresh basil in her hummus. Not exactly Middle Eastern, but really tasty. Howard sometimes adds grated carrot or scallion to lighten the dish.

Scrambled Tofu

I love this dish—and any variation on it—because it is quick, simple, and yet totally pleasing.

- 2 tablespoons extra-virgin olive oil
- 1 medium red onion, diced
- ½ teaspoon umeboshi vinegar
- 1 3-inch piece burdock, sliced into matchsticks
- 1 medium carrot, sliced into matchsticks
- 6–8 fresh button mushrooms, sliced
- 1 pound firm or extra-firm tofu
- 1–2 tablepoons shoyu
- Kernels from 1 ear corn
- 1 teaspoon curry or chile powder (optional)
- ¼–½ cup spring water
- ¼ cup chopped scallions, cilantro, or parsley for garnish

Heat the oil in a skillet over medium heat. Add onion and sauté for about 1 minute. Sprinkle the umeboshi vinegar on the onion, which helps it to keeps its reddish color. Sauté until the onion is soft. Add burdock and sauté a few minutes, then add the carrot and sauté for a few more minutes. Add mushrooms and sauté until they are soft. With your hands, crumble the tofu into the skillet. Add the shoyu, corn, spices, and enough of the spring water to wet the bottom of the pan. Cover, allowing the whole mixture to steam for about 3–5 minutes over low heat. Remove from heat, toss with garnish, and serve.

SERVES 4

Variation
Try this with any vegetable you like that sautés well. *Mmmmm.*

Black-Eyed Pea Croquettes

This is another most excellent recipe invented by my friend Lisa Silverman. This dish is quick, easy, and really, really yummy. I'm so lucky I live right down the street from her.

- 2 cups black-eyed peas, soaked overnight in spring water
- ½ teaspoon sea salt
- 1 tablespoon shoyu
- 1 teaspoon ground cumin
- 2 cups safflower oil for frying

Dipping Sauce
- ½ cup barley malt
- 1–2 tablespoons organic Dijon mustard
- Chopped parsley or cilantro for garnish

Place soaked beans in food processor. Add salt, shoyu, and cumin. Blend until you get fine shreds of bean, but don't blend into a pulp. The mixture will be slightly wet but can hold together. Form palm-sized croquettes with your hands. Heat 1 inch of oil in a cast-iron skillet to about 350°F. To test the oil, drop in a tiny amount of croquette mixture. If it bubbles furiously and rises to the top, the oil is ready. Do not let the oil get so hot that it smokes. You may need to make little adjustments to the heat under the oil throughout the cooking process to avoid burning the croquettes. Place 4 croquettes in the oil and let fry for about 4 minutes on each side. Place on paper towel to drain extra oil. Heat barley malt and mustard over low heat until it bubbles. Pour over croquettes or into individual dipping bowls. Garnish with parsley or cilantro. Serve while still hot.

**MAKES 12 MEDIUM-SIZED CROQUETTES,
WHICH SERVES 4**

Variation
Blend ½ cup chopped cilantro or parsley in the food processor with the beans and skip the garnish.

Corn Pona Lisa (Black Bean and Corn Bread Casserole)

Another excellent recipe by Lisa. Come to Maine and take her classes!

- 2 cups dried black turtle beans, soaked overnight with 2-inch piece kombu
- 2 tablespoons olive oil
- 1 large onion, diced
- 1 clove garlic, minced
- ½ teaspoon sea salt
- Kernels from 4 ears corn
- 1 teaspoon ground cumin
- 1 tablespoon ginger juice
- 2 tablespoons shoyu
- ¼ cup chopped fresh cilantro
- Corn or olive oil

Corn Bread

- 2½ cups cornmeal
- 1½ cups whole-wheat pastry flour
- 1⅓ cups unbleached white flour
- 3 tablespoons baking powder
- 1 teaspoon sea salt
- 1¼ cups water
- 1⅓ cups soy milk
- ⅔ cup light olive oil
- ½ cup maple syrup
- ½ teaspoon vanilla extract

Preheat oven to 400°F. After beans and kombu have soaked, discard the soaking water. Slice kombu into thin strips. Place beans and kombu in a 4- or 5-liter pressure cooker and cover with fresh water so that the water comes up about 1 inch over the beans. Close the pressure cooker and bring the beans to pressure. Place flame deflector under pressure cooker, reduce heat to medium-low, and cook 30 minutes (if you don't have a pressure cooker, cook beans in a saucepan with kombu over medium-low heat for 1½ hours).

While beans are cooking, heat olive oil in a skillet over medium heat. Sauté onions, garlic, sea salt, and corn until onions are translucent, about 5 minutes. Grate a 2-inch piece of ginger into a pulp and then squeeze out 1 tablespoon of juice. Add cumin, ginger juice, and shoyu, and cook for another 5 minutes. When beans are cooked, strain them and add to onion mixture. Mix in cilantro. Pour mixture into a lightly oiled 9-by-13-inch casserole dish—use corn or olive oil.

For corn bread topping: sift together dry ingredients and then blend together wet ingredients. Mix them together until just blended.

Pour batter over black-bean mixture and bake for 40–45 minutes. Let cool at least 15 minutes before serving.

SERVES 6

sea vegetables

When I first started taking macrobiotic cooking classes, they still called this stuff "seaweed," which I loved, because I have a pet peeve about euphemisms. However, I suppose "seaweed" freaked too many people out, stopping them from making the transition to these INCREDIBLE foods, which is a shame, because seaweeds are truly that. Okay, not incredible necessarily like a cream-cheese-frosted carrot cake, but incredible like health food's SECRET WEAPON.

Sea vegetables have lots and lots of minerals: for example, they all have calcium, iron, phosphorus, potassium, manganese, sodium, zinc, and iodine. They have much higher mineral contents than land vegetables and all dairy products. And the extra bonus is that their minerals are all absorbable. They also include vitamins like A, C, and the Bs. We need minerals for our bones, skin, nails, hair, and many other functions in the body, and sea veggies are one of the best ways to get them.

Sea vegetables are antinuke: whoah. Sea veggies actually bind with radioactive substances in the body and release them. People living near Hiroshima and Nagasaki who ate sea vegetables did much better than those who didn't.

Sea vegetables keep our blood strong: blood is like the salty sea inside of us. Sea vegetables support the alkalinity that our blood should maintain for good health.

Sea vegetables soften us from the inside out: we look pretty dry from the outside, but we're kinda wet on the inside. Aging is basically about going from grape to raisin, and sea vegetables keep you young and juicy! Sea vegetables help us to maintain our inner fluids in a balanced way, helping with water metabolism and cleansing lymph fluid. They are also used to reduce many kinds of inflammation and have been known to soften hard masses in the body.

Sea vegetables should be used regularly, but in moderation: don't get all North American on me and think that now, since you've found the perfect food, you should eat four pounds of it every day. Remember yin and yang: extreme yin becomes extreme yang, so we can never afford to get extreme unless we want to create imbalances. We can get too many minerals, which leads to its own set of problems. So don't go crazy. In macrobiotic cooking, sea vegetables are found in soups and bean dishes and are added to other vegetable dishes. To get all the great benefits of sea veggies, cook an arame or hijiki dish once a week. And try to eat half a sheet of nori every day.

The types of seaweeds used regularly in macrobiotic cooking are:

- *Agar agar:* these blond little flakes are added to liquid to make gels, like puddings or aspics.
- *Arame:* consisting of thin, dark shreds, arame is usually sautéed with vegetables as a side dish.
- *Dulse:* a reddish sea vegetable used in soups and condiments, it is very high in protein.
- *Hijiki:* the strongest sea vegetable, hijiki comes dried in long or short "strings" and has the most fishy flavor. It needs to be reconstituted before cooking. It is best sautéed with other vegetables. You may have had hijiki in a seaweed salad at a Japanese restaurant (although it's usually cooked with sugar!).
- *Kombu:* Japanese kelp. Kombu is soaked and used in bean dishes to make them more digestible and to add minerals. It can also be added to grains, instead of salt, and in broth for noodles or nabe vegetables. Kombu is always placed at the bottom of the pot for nishime vegetables and can be boiled or roasted to be put into a homemade condiment.
- *Nori:* any maki roll in a sushi restaurant is made with nori sea vegetable. Pressed into sheets, it tastes best lightly toasted and can be eaten as is, rolled as sushi or cooked into a condiment.
- *Wakame:* this is the green stuff floating around in miso soup. It can also be cooked with vegetables and beans, pressed into pressed salads, or baked and ground into a condiment.

All Hail Hijiki

Hijiki is the alpha male of sea vegetables. Loaded with minerals, it packs a serious nutritional punch and is incredibly good for your hair, nails, skin, and bones. In fact, after eating a serving of this dish, I notice that my skin feels softer immedi-

ately. Hijiki also has a fishy flavor, so it may take some getting used to. If this dish is too strong for you, substitute arame, which is a little milder in taste and intensity.

- Medium handful dried hijiki, soaked in spring water for 30 minutes
- 2 tablespoons toasted sesame oil
- 1 onion, sliced into half-moons
- Pinch sea salt
- Spring water
- 1 tablespoon shoyu
- 1 tablespoon mirin
- 1 medium carrot, sliced into matchsticks
- Scallions for garnish

While hijiki is soaking in spring water, chop the vegetables. When the hijiki is softened, discard the soaking water and, if the hijiki is in long strands, chop it into 1-inch pieces. Most companies, however, sell hijiki in little strands. Heat the sesame oil over a medium flame in a heavy skillet that has a lid. Add the onion and sauté for a few minutes, adding the salt. Add the hijiki and sauté it with the onion, coating it lightly in oil. Add water to halfway up the hijiki and onion. Bring to a boil and add shoyu and mirin. Cover and let simmer 30 minutes. Add carrot matchsticks on top. Let simmer 10 more minutes. Garnish with scallions.

SERVES 4

Variation

To do this recipe using arame instead of hijiki, simply rinse arame (no soaking required) and reduce cooking time by 10 minutes. Feel free to use light sesame or olive oil for seasonal variety. This recipe is delicious with fresh corn, snow peas, green beans, or any vegetable that rocks your boat.

Baked Wakame with Onion and Squash

This dish rules.

- 2 cups onion, sliced in thin half-moons
- 1 cup wakame, soaked and sliced into 2-inch pieces (reserve soaking water for use in recipe)
- 2 tablespoons sesame tahini
- 1 teaspoon shoyu
- ½ small buttercup or butternut squash, thinly sliced (unpeeled if organic)

Preheat oven to 350°F. Place onion in a saucepan with a small amount of wakame soaking water. Bring to boil, cover, reduce flame, and simmer for 5 minutes. Remove and place in a small casserole dish. Mix wakame with onion. Dilute tahini with about ½ cup wakame soaking water and shoyu. Mix with wakame and onion. Smooth mixture evenly in casserole dish, and layer sliced squash over the top till covered. Cover and bake in oven for 30 minutes. Remove cover and bake another 10–15 minutes to remove excess liquid and slightly brown top.

SERVES 4–6

Arame Tofu Dumplings

Lisa Silverman thought this up as a creative way to get seaweed into her daughter, Ella. It works.

- 1-pound block tofu, pressed for 10 minutes
- 1-inch piece ginger, peeled and grated
- ½ cup soaked arame
- 2 tablespoons umeboshi vinegar
- 2 tablespoons shoyu
- 1 tablespoon mirin
- 2 scallions, finely chopped
- Dumpling wrappers (available in most health-food stores—try to get the ones without eggs)
- Sesame or safflower oil for frying

Crumble tofu and mix in next six ingredients. Place 1 heaping tablespoon in each dumpling wrapper, then fold in half to make a triangle. Wet edges of wrapper and press together all around to seal. Coat skillet generously with oil. Fry each dumpling on both sides in a covered skillet until golden brown. Place on paper towels. Serve with Tempura Dip Sauce (see p. 197).

MAKES APPROXIMATELY 18 DUMPLINGS

Variation

Try adding some tahini or peanut butter to make them even yummier to kids.

soups

Basic Miso Soup

There are a million permutations to basic miso soup—experiment with different misos and different vegetables. The only consistent elements of miso soup are water, wakame, and miso. Everything else changes. This is a very simple and traditional recipe that can act as a springboard for your future soupfests.

- 2-inch piece of dried wakame
- 2 dried shiitake mushrooms
- 5 cups spring water
- ½ medium onion, sliced into half-moons
- 1 inch daikon, thinly sliced
- 4 teaspoons barley miso, aged at least 2 years
- 1 scallion, thinly sliced for garnish

Soak wakame and shiitake mushrooms in 1 cup of the spring water for 10 minutes. Cut the thick wakame stem away from the soft "frond." If it is not too tough, slice the stem into tiny pieces and the rest of the wakame into bite-sized pieces. Remove and discard the tough stems of the shiitakes and slice the caps into thin strips. In a saucepan, bring the spring water (4 remaining cups), wakame, shiitake, onion, and soaking water to a boil. Reduce heat and let simmer 10 minutes.

Remove about ¼ cup of the broth and add the miso to it. Using a suribachi and surikogi (or a spoon), puree the miso until it is smoothly integrated into the broth. Pour the miso liquid back into the soup. Let it simmer for 3 more minutes. Do not let it come to a boil—that will overcook the live enzymes. Serve in individual bowls and garnish with sliced scallion.

MAKES 4 SERVINGS

Variations

Oil-sauté onion and thinly sliced winter squash before adding water and wakame. Finish with light miso and fresh corn kernels. Garnish with parsley.

Other options: cauliflower and fresh mushrooms. Onions, summer squash, and tofu.

Once in a while, add burdock to make your miso soup nice and strengthening.

Squeeze some ginger juice into the soup at the end to make it more dynamic.

Bake tiny cubes of mochi and float them in the soup as croutons.

Regularly add fresh greens like watercress or bok choy to the miso at the end of cooking.

Mushroom Barley Soup

- 8 button mushrooms, sliced
- ½ cup barley, best soaked in spring water overnight
- 6 cups spring water
- 1-inch piece kombu
- 3 thin slices ginger
- 2 tablespoons olive oil
- 2 medium onions, diced
- 3 tablespoons rolled oats or brown rice flour
- 2½ tablespoons barley miso or to taste
- 1 teaspoon lemon juice (optional)
- Fresh watercress or parsley for garnish

Place mushrooms, barley, water, kombu, and ginger in a pot. Bring to a boil and simmer 40 minutes or until barley is softened. With a handheld food processor, whiz the rolled oats into almost a flour.

Heat the oil in a skillet over medium heat and sauté the onions. Add the flour and sauté with onions, coating them well. Take ½ cup of soup from the pot and slowly stir it into onion-flour mixture, avoiding lumping. Add to soup mixture.

Dilute miso in a cup with some of the soup. Add this liquid to the soup and let simmer 5 minutes. Right at the end, squeeze the lemon juice, if desired, into the soup. Garnish and serve.

SERVES 4–6

Variation

Feel free to build on this soup with corn kernels, diced celery, and roasted red pepper toward the end.

Corn Chowdah

- 6 ears corn
- 1 2-inch strip kombu
- 6–8 cups spring water
- 1 teaspoon corn oil
- 1 large onion, diced
- 1 leek, thinly sliced
- 2 medium carrots, diced
- ½ cup cornmeal
- 1–2 tablespoons white miso or sea salt to taste
- Fresh chopped dill or basil for garnish

Slice corn off cob with a sharp knife. Place cobs and kombu in medium-sized pot. Add water, bring to a boil, and simmer 15 minutes. In a large soup pot, heat corn oil and sauté onion and leek until onion is translucent. Add carrots and sauté 3 more minutes. Add corn and sauté 1 more minute. Sprinkle cornmeal into pot and stir well until vegetables are coated. When mixture begins to turn golden, strain cobs from stock and add stock to soup pot, stirring quickly to prevent lumps.

Place on flame deflector and simmer for 30 minutes. Dissolve miso or sea salt and simmer for 3–4 minutes. Use chopped fresh dill or chopped fresh basil for garnish.

SERVES 6–8

Squash Soup

Great squash soup is all about the squash. During the late summer and autumn, squash hits its peak of sweetness and you have a variety to choose from: hokkaido pumpkin, buttercup, and butternut all make great soup. Delicata, one of the sweetest, is a little more difficult to deskin, but if you have the patience, go for it. This dish is soothing, imparts good-quality sweetness, and—because it is nourishing to the pancreas—is very centering and stabilizing.

- 4–6 cups winter squash, seeded, peeled (optional), and cut into 2-inch chunks
- 1 2-inch piece dried kombu
- Spring water
- ½ teaspoon sea salt

or

- 2 tablespoons white miso

or

- 2 tablespoons shoyu
- Chopped scallion, parsley, or cilantro for garnish

Place the squash and kombu in a 6-quart pot and add water to just cover the squash. (For a thinner soup, use more water.) Cover and bring to a boil. Simmer 30 minutes. Puree in a hand food mill, blender, or by using a handheld food processor in the soup. Return soup to pot and add seasoning. Simmer 10 more minutes. Garnish with scallion, cilantro, or parsley and serve.

SERVES 4–6

Split-Pea Soup

My stepgrandfather, George, used to make split-pea soup when I was a kid. The joke in the family was the first prize was a bowl of George's soup, and second prize was two bowls. So it's funny that I like split-pea soup so much now. But hey, everything eventually becomes its opposite! The secret to this recipe is the burdock, which imparts a nice smoky taste like ham.

- 2 cups green or yellow split peas
- 10–12 cups spring water, depending on the thickness you desire
- 2 inches wakame, soaked 5 minutes
- 1 medium red onion, in large dices
- 1 medium burdock root, diced
- 1–2 cups winter squash, in bite-sized chunks
- 1 cup leeks, sliced in about ½-inch slices on the diagonal
- 2–3 tablespoons white miso
- 1 tablespoon shoyu
- 1 tablespoon lemon juice (optional)
- Scallions or parsley for garnish

Sort and wash the split peas carefully. Cut the wakame from its tough stems and chop into 1-inch squares. In a 6-quart pot, bring water, wakame, and split peas to a boil. Skim off any foam that comes to the surface. Add onion, burdock, and squash. Boil for 2 minutes, then cover and simmer for 40 minutes. Add leeks, and simmer 10 more minutes. For a really creamy soup, take about 3–4 cups of soup and puree it in a blender, then return it to the pot. In a cup or suribachi, dilute miso with a little soup and mix it well until creamy. Add miso and shoyu to soup. Let simmer 4 minutes. Add lemon juice, if desired, and garnish.

SERVES 6–8

Variation

For an even heartier, meatier taste, add a generous pinch of dried bonito flakes during the last 10 minutes of cooking.

Noodles in Broth

- 1 8-ounce package udon or soba noodles
- A 3-inch strip kombu

- 2 dried shiitake mushrooms, soaked in 1 cup water for 15 minutes, destemmed, and sliced
- 4 cups spring water
- 2–3 tablespoons shoyu
- 1 tablespoon mirin (optional)
- 1 drop brown rice vinegar (optional)
- Scallions for garnish
- 1 sheet toasted nori sea vegetable, cut into 1-inch-by-¼-inch strips
- Toasted sesame seeds, bonito flakes, or grated ginger (optional)

Cook noodles, rinse with cold water, and drain. Place kombu and shiitake in a pot and add water and shiitake soaking water. Bring to a boil. Reduce flame to medium-low and simmer for about 10 minutes. Remove kombu and slice into thin strips and add back to the stock. Reduce the flame to low. Add shoyu (add mirin and vinegar, if desired) to taste and simmer for 3–5 minutes. Place the noodles in serving bowls and ladle broth on top of them. Garnish with scallions, slices of shiitake, and strips of nori. If desired, add optional garnishes, too.

SERVES 4

Variation
Use cabbage, onions, squash, carrots, broccoli, or other vegetables in the broth.

pickles

Red Radish Umeboshi Pickles

Note: this recipe can be used with carrots, onions, broccoli, cauliflower, daikon, turnip, or any other relatively hearty vegetable. And you can pickle a bunch of vegetables in one jar together.

- 6 red radishes, washed and thinly sliced
- ½ cup umeboshi vinegar
- 1 cup spring water

Place the radish slices in a Pyrex cup or mason jar. Pour the liquid over them (no matter the amount, this brine ratio is 1 part vinegar to 2 parts water). Cover the container with gauze or cheesecloth and secure with a rubber band. Pickles need air in order for fermentation to take place. Put the jar in a room-temperature, unhurried place in the kitchen and let pickle for one day. Take out one-third of the pickles, rinse them off with a little water, eat some, and keep the rest refrigerated.

After two days, take out some more and rinse. After three days, remove the remaining pickles and rinse. Now you have three different strengths of pickle to satisfy the whole family. Umeboshi pickles are rarely pickled more than three days.

MAKES 12 SERVINGS

Variation

Do this recipe the same way using shoyu instead of umeboshi vinegar.

Miso Pickles

These are fun and very easy.

- A variety of root vegetables
- A crock or jar full of miso

Wash the vegetables under water, scrubbing with a vegetable brush. Let them sit, whole, in a cool, shady place for about a day, or until they soften a little. Ideally, you should be able to bend the vegetable into a curve. If you are pickling the whole vegetable, cut a number of slits into each root.

Otherwise, cut them into medium-thick diagonal slices. Place the vegetables in the miso so that they are completely covered.

The sliced vegetables will be done in three to seven days, and whole vegetables will take one to two weeks. Rinse before serving and take only small amounts, for these pickles are very strong.

desserts

Kanten (Pudding)

Don't forget the fruit kanten with creamy topping on page 139. Kantens are regular "whole hog" desserts.

Mochazake Pie

Being an inveterate chocolate lover, I am always looking for delicious macrobiotic yummies that simulate versions of my old pal cocoa. Re-creating a mocha flavor, this recipe is best when made with Kendall's amasake (which isn't distributed nationally in retail outlets but can be delivered to your door), although amasake from the health-food store is fine, too. Feel free to adjust the nut butter and grain coffee ratios to strike your personal fancy. You can also experiment with different crusts or serve this dish simply as a pudding.

Pie Crust
- 1½ cups whole-wheat pastry flour
- ¼ teaspoon sea salt

- ¼ cup safflower oil
- ¼ cold apple juice

Preheat oven to 375°F. Combine flour, salt, and oil together, mashing with a fork. When mixed together, slowly add the apple juice to create a dough. Knead the ball of dough for a few minutes. Roll the dough between two sheets of wax paper to make a circle approximately 10 inches in diameter. Lay the circle in a prepared 9-inch pie tin. Prick the dough liberally with a fork. Cover the pie tin with aluminum foil, laying it right against the dough and folding it over the sides of the crust. Bake for 15 minutes. Remove foil and bake for 5 more minutes. Set aside to cool.

Filling
- 1 quart plain amasake (set aside ¼ cup for diluting kuzu)
- ½ cup hazelnut butter
- 2 tablespoons grain coffee
- 1 teaspoon umeboshi vinegar
- ½ teaspoon vanilla (optional)
- 3 level tablespoons agar agar flakes
- 2 tablespoons kuzu
- 2 tablespoons roasted hazelnuts for garnish
- ¼ teaspoon grain coffee for garnish

Blend first five ingredients in a blender until smooth. Pour into a saucepan, stir in agar agar, and bring to a boil over a medium flame. Reduce the flame to low and let simmer 15 minutes, whisking regularly to prevent sticking and also to help the agar agar dissolve. Be sure to cook it the full 15 minutes, even if it appears that the agar agar has dissolved. If you don't cook it long enough, the undissolved agar agar can haunt you as tiny tapiocalike balls after the filling has set. Dilute kuzu in cold amasake and add to pot. Stir constantly to avoid lumps. Bring to a boil again, then back to a simmer. After about a minute, the mixture should thicken slightly. Pour into prepared pie crust and let set. Garnish and serve.

SERVES 8

Pears with Ginger Glaze and Pecan Cream

Pecan Cream
- 2 cups pecans
- 1 cup soy milk
- ¼ cup rice syrup
- 2 teaspoons vanilla extract
- ½ teaspoon umeboshi vinegar

Pears
- 4 pears, preferably Bosc, peeled, cored, and halved
- 2 cups pear juice (set aside ¼ cup for diluting kuzu)
- 1 teaspoon ginger juice
- 1 tablespoon kuzu
- 8 sprigs fresh mint for garnish

Preheat oven to 350°F. Place pecans on cookie sheet and bake 10 minutes. Transfer toasted pecans to food processor and grind into a powder. Transfer remaining cream ingredients into a blender and blend until smooth. Refrigerate for 30 minutes.

Place pears in 6-quart pot. Add pear juice and ginger juice. Bring to a boil, then cover, reduce heat, and simmer for about 10 minutes, or until pears are soft. Remove pears and place in individual serving dishes. Thicken the leftover juice in bottom of pot with diluted kuzu, stirring constantly to avoid lumping. Pour kuzu glaze over pears, add a dollop of pecan cream, and garnish with a sprig of fresh mint.

SERVES 8

Really Yummy Oat Bars

- ½ cup whole-wheat flour
- 1½ cups rolled oats
- 1 teaspoon cinnamon
- ½ teaspoon nutmeg
- ½ teaspoon baking soda*
- ¼ teaspoon sea salt
- ⅓ cup maple syrup
- ⅓ cup corn oil
- ½ teaspoon vanilla
- ⅓ cup unsweetened fruit spread

Preheat oven to 350°F. In a bowl, mix the dry ingredients. Add maple syrup, corn oil, and vanilla, mixing thoroughly. In a small baking pan or Pyrex dish, press half the mixture like a thick pie crust. Spread the fruit jam onto it and cover with the rest of the oat mixture. Bake for 25 minutes. Although you should let this dessert cool before cutting into bars, it's not that easy.

MAKES 6 SMALL BARS

---

* Baking soda is generally not used in macrobiotic cooking, but I couldn't help myself—this recipe is so good!

Seaweed Nut Crunch

Many thanks to Amy Rolnick for letting me use this recipe. It has saved me lots of money on snacks at the health-food store.

- ⅓ cup corn oil
- ½ cup maple syrup
- 1 cup sliced almonds
- 1 cup sesame seeds
- 6 sheets nori seaweed, torn into little pieces
- 1 teaspoon shoyu or to taste

Preheat oven to 350°F. Pour corn oil and maple syrup in a large skillet. Bring to a frothy boil and add sliced almonds, stir, and add sesame seeds and nori pieces. Sprinkle in shoyu. Continue stirring until everything is coated. Pour into one layer on a baking sheet. Bake for 10 minutes. Let cool and enjoy.

SERVES 6

Apple-Blueberry Crisp

- 6 Cortland or MacIntosh apples
- 1 quart blueberries, cleaned
- 3 cups apple juice (and 1 cup for diluting kuzu)
- 6 tablespoons kuzu
- 1 teaspoon umeboshi vinegar
- 2 teaspoons vanilla
- Pinch sea salt

Topping
- 3 cups oats
- 2 cups barley flour
- ¾ cup corn oil
- ¾ cup rice syrup
- ¼ maple syrup
- 1 cup chopped walnuts or pecans

- ¼ teaspoon sea salt
- ¼ teaspoon cinnamon

Preheat oven to 350°F. Slice apples and place them in a 9-by-12-inch baking pan with blueberries. Heat apple juice. When it's hot, add diluted kuzu and vinegar, stirring continually to avoid lumping. Bring to boil and let simmer for 2 minutes. Turn off heat and add vanilla.

In a skillet over medium-low heat, dry-roast the oats, barley flour, salt, and cinnamon for about 5 minutes. Heat oil and syrup together. Pour over flour mixture and mix well. Add nuts. Pour apple juice mixture over apples and blueberries. Cover with oat/rice-syrup mixture. Cover with tinfoil and bake for 30 minutes. Remove foil and bake 15–25 minutes more. Let cool for about 30 minutes before serving.

SERVES 8–12

Couscous Cake

This is a great recipe to make at the beginning of the week and then just have sitting around for snacks. Because it's not baked, it is an appropriate dessert for any season and is quite relaxing. The topping on its own makes a really delicious treat.

Cake
- 2 cups apple juice
- 2 tablespoons rice syrup
- 1 teaspoon vanilla
- ½ teaspoon umeboshi vinegar
- 1 cup whole-wheat couscous

Topping
- 1 cup dried fruit (prunes, apples, apricots, raisins)
- 1 cup apple juice

- 1 cup spring water
- 2 tablespoons rice syrup
- ½ teaspoon vanilla
- ½ teaspoon umeboshi vinegar
- 2 strips lemon zest
- 1 tablespoon kuzu
- ¼ cup cold water

Bring the apple juice, rice syrup, vanilla, and vinegar to a boil. Add the couscous and let simmer over a low flame for 5 minutes. Remove from heat and let sit 20 minutes. Place the couscous in 9-by-9-inch dish and tamp it down to make the "cake."

Topping: soak dried fruit in apple juice for 30 minutes. Chopped soaked fruit in bite-sized pieces. Bring soaked fruit, soaking juice, and water to a boil. Add rice syrup, vanilla, umeboshi vinegar, and lemon zest. Cover and let simmer about 15 minutes. Dilute kuzu in the cold water, mixing well to smooth out any lumps. Stir kuzu dilution into fruit, stirring constantly. Let this come to a boil for 1 minute, then remove from heat. Remove lemon zest from topping. Spread topping on couscous cake. Let it cool and serve.

SERVES 4

condiments

Condiments are a big deal in macrobiotics. A great way to get good-quality minerals to the blood, they are also an easy way to overuse salt, which can make a woman tight and irritable. Salt is the strongest agent of contraction in any diet, and because of its Japanese heritage, the macrobiotic diet can lean in the salty direction. The point here being: go easy on the condiments. Between ½ and 1 teaspoon of gomashio a day is ample, and just a tiny sprinkling of the others.

There are some good condiments available at the health-food store, like tekka, Eden shake, and shiso sprinkle. Try them. However, it's important to make your own fresh condiments, like the two that follow, since crushed sesame seeds become rancid quite quickly, and the quality of the salt you use will be better than a commercial brand.

Gomashio

Gomashio (from "goma" for sesame and "shio" for salt) is the most popular and regularly used condiment, and it is very easy to make. The yin of the sesame oil and the yang of the salt make a very nice balance that is especially supportive of heart function. Gomashio gets stale after a couple of weeks, so be sure to make it fresh regularly.

- 1 teaspoon sea salt
- 18 teaspoons black or tan sesame seeds

In a stainless-steel or cast-iron skillet, roast the sea salt over medium heat. Keep it moving in the skillet and roast it until 1) it becomes a sort of an off-white color and 2) it emits an ammonialike smell. This should take about 3 minutes. Place the roasted salt in a suribachi.*

Rinse the sesame seeds in a strainer and place them in a skillet over medium heat. Move them constantly until they dry off. Reduce heat to low and continue to stir regularly until most of the seeds have popped or have puffed up a little. Be careful not to let them burn. In the suribachi, grind the salt with a the surikogi until it no longer has any large granules. It should be a fine powder.

Add the roasted sesame seeds and grind until about 75 percent of the seeds are cracked open. This may take about 5–10 minutes of grinding,

---

*A suribachi may be your first macro kitchen purchase. It is a serrated bowl that comes with a wooden pestle called a surikogi. They can be found at most health-food stores or ordered from macro suppliers. They are cheap and really the most perfect tool for doing this job.

but the smell is amazing, and you can pass it along to kids or others in the kitchen. Everyone likes making gomashio.

If you stick to 1 teaspoon of gomashio a day, this batch should last one person just over two weeks.

18 SERVINGS

Nori Condiment

This one looks yucky but tastes great. It is wonderful served with rice or other grains (serving size is 1 teaspoon) and keeps in the fridge for up to a week.

- 5 sheets nori
- Spring water
- ½ teaspoon mirin
- 1½ teaspoons shoyu
- ½ teaspoon grated ginger

Rip or break nori into squares and place in a saucepan with water to just cover. Add the mirin and bring to a boil. Reduce flame to low and cover, letting it simmer until most of the water has cooked off and the nori forms a thick paste. Add the shoyu and the ginger. Simmer 5 minutes longer. Serve and keep the remainder refrigerated.

12 SERVINGS

CHAPTER NINE

beyond the diet: desludging and the yin and yang of love

B y being macrobiotic, it's as if you're going backward. You begin to look younger, feel younger, and a lifetime of accumulation is released from your body. As this desludging takes place, it begins to become very clear where and how your energy is moving. Life becomes more about the vibrational world than the material world. In this chapter, we will discuss the phenomenon of desludging, as well as consider all the ways your fresh, strong life force can move. Some of the most basic expressions of human energy are love and sexuality. We finish the chapter by exploring the yin and yang of love.

desludging

I had been macrobiotic for about six months in a really strict way. Before that, I had been eating good-quality, whole foods for about three years. I felt great, enjoying more energy than I had remembered since childhood. My life was smooth, changing, healing all the time. Therapy was going well, and old issues were coming up and poofing away in puffs of smoke. It was cool.

Then one day, after walking up the five flights to my East Village apartment, I aimed the key at the lock in my door and it missed the target. I tried again. It was still a little off, but I could slide it into the hole from the left. "That's weird," I thought, as I entered the apartment and dumped the groceries on the kitchen table. But it being the only clue that day that something was askew, I let it slip from my consciousness.

The next day the key was even wilier. It was as if the electronic circuitry of my nervous system had been messed with in the night. I got scared. I sat down in my apartment and tried to go over the million normal things this could be—multiple sclerosis, tiny strokes, Parkinson's—just to calm myself down. Suddenly, I felt a pulsing in my foot. Not a blood-type pulse, but a lightninglike shiver as little bolts of electricity seemed to exit my foot. Something was definitely up. I had never experienced any of this before, and surely I was going to die. But first, I would crumple up into a wheelchair and petrify like a conch shell.

Hoping like hell that this nightmare would wrap itself up spontaneously, I avoided going to a doctor. I was only twenty-six and I had never had any significant health problems, so I was far from hypochondriacal. In fact, the anxiety that accompanied this mysterious condition seemed unusual to me, almost as if it were a part of the package. A physical instability creating an emotional instability. Eschewing the medical route for a few days, I tried the folk remedy of sharing excessively with all my friends, freaking them out with conversations like this:

ME: ultra-serious, staring into my tea: "I need to tell you something."

FRIEND: reaching out across restaurant table to take my hand. "What is it, Jess?"

ME: "It's gonna sound weird." Looking at FRIEND with scared, puppy-dog eyes.

FRIEND: "Yeah?"

ME: "Well . . . I've been having this shaking and pulsing in my hands and feet, and I don't know what it is, but (voice cracking up) I'm pretty sure I'm headed for a wheelchair, and I just hope you'll be there for me." Crying ensues.

Finally, my friend Janet forced me to go to her beloved Doctor Silverman. With an office on Central Park West, this guy was the real deal. What I needed now was not an acupuncturist, or a nutritionist, not even Michio Kushi himself. I needed a guy, preferably a really smart guy, with a bunch of letters after his name, to whom I would pay $375 for him to look me up and down, hammer at my knees, peer in my ears, and tell me I was okay.

By the time I booked the appointment and got in to see him, the symptoms had lessened somewhat. Although he wasn't sure exactly what was going on, he could assure me, from all his expensive education, that it was not the big nasties I had anticipated; as far as he could tell, there was no wheelchair on the horizon. Tears of gratitude now.

The only quasi-satisfactory answer I got was from another macrobiotic person who said that anyone following the macrobiotic diet can go through some pretty terrific (and terrifying) shifts. "It's just a discharge," she said, like every other macro I had ever known, as if they were describing a light rain shower over Topeka.

The proof was in the pudding when the symptoms never returned. Nor did the weird shin pain I had for a few days, or the horrendous diarrhea. I even needed glasses for about a year, never having been bespectacled before, and then, when my body balanced out, I threw them away!

As the body surrenders to the scrubbing bubbles of organic whole foods, prepared in a balanced way respecting yin and yang, all the yuck and dirt and sludge of the past comes up and out. That's discharge. It can be mucus, a rash, weird dreams, zits, aches and pains, drug flashbacks, or any number of other funky releases. But the point is, it's stuff coming out, and as long as you continue to eat whole grains and vegetables, refraining from sludgy foods, you can be sure that weird symptoms are simply discharge.

After a discharge, one feels lighter and freer. But discharges themselves, especially at the beginning, can feel bad. When I was the manager of the "Way to Health" program at the Kushi Institute, every week a new crew of about a dozen people would check in on Sunday night. They were fed meal after meal of some of the best macrobiotic food available: organic brown rice, hulled that day. Pure local well water from the Berkshire Mountains. Organic vegetables grown on the property. And the food was prepared by experienced, loving cooks. After most meals, the participants would go outside and take a walk in the most oxygen-rich air they had breathed in years. Put this all together and basically we had roto-rooters going through their bodies.

The cycle of discharge was consistent week to week: on Monday, everyone was sort of shy and reserved, most people retreating to their rooms for a nap in the afternoon. By Tuesday, the headaches came crashing down—not only on the big coffee drinkers, but the sugar lovers were all suffering from being contracted so fast and hard. Everyone was moody. By Wednesday, there was downright irritability and depression, but no one wanted to admit it.

But Thursday morning, every Thursday morning, was like Christmas and

Passover and New Year's all wrapped into one. People bouncing into early-morning exercise class greeting each other like old high-school buddies. They declared they hadn't slept so well in years! Pains in the head and neck and shoulders were *gone*. Decade-old rashes had disappeared in the night. A weird joy was bubbling up out of nowhere. And the sunrise looked so damned *beautiful!*

Most profound was the transition made by the cynical spouses, the ones who had been dragged up into the mountain to support their ill mates. I'm sure they loved their partners very much, but come on, a lifetime of birdseed and tofu is pushing it. Because they expected nothing from this ride except misery, they were the most amazed and impressed and delighted by the Thursday morning feeling. Extreme yang becomes yin. By noon, they were tooling around the store throwing pressure cookers and sushi mats into the shopping cart saying, "Come on, honey, you need this and this and this!" What they were experiencing was the first taste of real health. And, luckily, it is addictive.

If you're interested in experiencing discharges—in really desludging your body—go whole hog for six months to a year, keeping oily foods and flour products to a minimum. That will produce one of the most interesting years of your life. But to do that diet with some dairy, or some chocolate, or a little bacon or some coffee now and then will significantly reduce your body's ability to discharge. If sludge is being put in, discharge slows or stops. If deep discharge is to occur, sludge needs to be avoided completely. Now, very few people can practice the desludging diet perfectly, so if you stray, just get right back up in the saddle, but do your best.

As your body desludges, you could experience any or many of the following: constipation, diarrhea, headaches, cravings for old foods, irritability, depression, disturbed sleep, lack of sleep, lots of sleep, rashes and other skin conditions, nausea, weird aches and pains, phlegm, hair loss, drug flashbacks, loss of menstrual flow, loss of libido (these last two occur because your life force is being called to your vital organs for cleanup, and nature considers your reproductive organs secondary to the vitals—sort of luxury organs—but it all comes back within a few months), plus any number of things I have forgotten. But that's only the funky stuff. You can also expect to feel peaceful, calm, light, silly, ridiculously happy for no reason, and tremendously excited about life itself. If any discharge or symptoms persist, it may be a good idea to consult a macrobiotic counselor for guidance.

The possibilities here are endless. Considering it takes seven years to regenerate every type of cell in the human body, if you were to start now, eating a balanced macrobiotic diet for seven years, you would be a completely different person—different blood, different consciousness, probably a different direction in life, one that supports you better as an individual, and the planet as a whole. Forget the migraines. Or the psoriasis. Or even the tumor. That stuff goes early. I'm talking about a complete life overhaul that includes every level of your being and your relationship to the universe itself. Cool.

Eating at fast-food restaurants every day for seven years will change your life, too—in the other direction. But your body makes a valiant attempt to handle it all: at first, sludge is dealt with through normal channels of discharge—urination, defecation, perspiration, and respiration. But sludge also comes out of us in the form of hopeless moods and negative thoughts. Sludge affects our relationships, not just sexually but emotionally. Most tragic perhaps is the way sludge can cut us off energetically from our source, the Infinite Universe and nature. We feel locked in, cut off, and the television actually begins to make sense.

If more sludge goes in and no natural stuff gets introduced to help kick the sludge out, it begins to take over the body. Suddenly pooping and peeing, breathing and sweating can't do the whole job: now stuff needs to creep out of the skin, in the form of acne and rashes and flakes. But sludge eventually catches up with the skin, too, mucking up the pores and creating a thickness that inhibits discharge; now sludge must collect beneath the skin. So layers of excess fat accrue around the organs. Excess fat and protein (sludge) within the organs are known as cysts or tumors. As the yucky energy gets deeper, the nervous system is affected and finally our spirit itself begins to die.

But seven years of accruing sludge is not that long. You may not notice any symptoms at all, because you're eating just like everybody else, looking just like everybody else, and feeling just like everybody else. You are like the lobster getting brought to a boil very, very slowly with all his buddies. But slow subcutaneous sludge accrual is the reason people show up for their yearly checkup and walk out with a terminal diagnosis. The body is so good at hiding problems, wanting so badly for you to enjoy the tennis game and the dinner party and the opera, that it packs away sludge as well as it can, feeling little or no compunction to alert you to its project. Poor thing. It is working on the naive and noble assumption that one day the sludge packing will stop and it will be able to get rid of all this crap.

Arrogance is basically ignoring or flouting the laws of nature. Until we harmonize with the yin and yang forces that are creating and uncreating us, we basically pack in more sludge, not even knowing that we're doing it. Or worse, we learn about sludge and reject the simple logic of it. This is the greatest arrogance of all. If you have read this far in this book and think it's all ridiculous, you are blind to your own spiritual sludge. It means that the simple laws of nature have not penetrated through your sludge armor. You may appear to be in great physical shape. You may have a beautiful tan. Perhaps you are very successful in the material world. Chances are you have a high IQ. But there is a type of energetic sludge that is holding you back from your true freedom and deepest happiness.

In what ways do you—as an individual—violate the order of the universe? Where are you packing sludge? Into your body? Into the environment? How much sludge can you pack into your life without feeling the effects? What do you realize you are currently "getting away with"? Considering yang becomes yin at its extreme, what may you be setting yourself up for?

where is your energy going?

After having desludged for a while, you will begin to perceive life as more of a vibrational event. As your body gets lighter, no longer weighed down or held back by excess fats, chemicals, and toxins, it's only natural to "tune in to" the lighter side of things—vibes. The Infinite Universe is pumping us full of vibrations every second of every day. And now that you are eating macrobiotically, respecting yin and yang, your physical vehicle—your body—will be stronger and feel more energized.

But health is not static. We don't get healthy just to sit around and feel good. We get healthy in order to live life thoroughly, and that vital energy we receive from the Infinite Universe needs to move outward into the world in order to stay bright and sparkly. So it's only natural that we get to the question "Where is your energy going?" In other words, how are you using your life force? Are you putting it into useful places, or is it being flushed down the energy toilet?

In this chapter we look at some of the many ways your energy moves into the world, how it can get "stuck," and how eating macrobiotically can free it to move in a more natural way. Let's begin with your head.

THINKING

Your brain is a thinking machine. But extreme foods can overcharge it or sludge it up so that it doesn't work as your friend. For example, sugar, caffeine, and other foods with extremely upward energy can drive an excess amount of energy into the head; you obsess about things, or spend the whole day in your head—at the expense of your other chakras. Because sugar also has a strongly expansive component, thoughts can literally expand right out of your head, making you spacy or scattered. Loss of minerals (yang) mean that it's hard to gather your thoughts or "get to the point" when conversing. Most people who jabber on and on, never really saying anything, have a sweet tooth or like to drink (yin).

Flour products make for cloudy thinking, and too much animal food can create rigidity in the mind as the arteries that feed the brain harden. Excess salt can yangize the mind so that it becomes closed and critical. But a brain fed natural, whole foods rich in minerals and good-quality carbohydrates is a beautiful thing.

First, the brain uses more blood sugar than any other organ in the body, so when you chew your grains and vegetables extremely well and those complex carbohydrates get delivered to the brain as natural blood sugar, your brain is very happy. Feelings of satisfaction, contentment, and peace flood the brain as it is bathed in natural sweetness. Good-quality minerals (found in whole grains, vegetables—but especially sea vegetables—and condiments) keep the blood slightly yang, which therefore attracts the yin world of vibrations and ideas. Great works of art, historical social advancements, and mind-blowing inventions all begin in the vibrational world as ideas or visions. It is our ability to pick up these vibrations and manifest them in the material world that determines whether they happen or not. A brain fed on natural, mineralized foods literally picks up information from the ether and has the stability and focus to give birth to those ideas as reality. So if you want to calm down the old brain a little, just sit down to a balanced macrobiotic meal and chew every mouthful one hundred times. You will be amazed at how peaceful and clear your mind becomes.

EMOTIONS

Are your emotions chaotic? Do they run your life? Are they so intense that they scare you? Do you have feelings at all? In Oriental medicine, feelings are connected to the internal organs. For instance, if someone is angry a lot, an acupuncturist thinks "*Hmm*. Liver/gall bladder energy is out of balance." So in the East, our feelings are an indicator of physical imbalance, and negative emotions are a sign that something is off-kilter in the body. And in macrobiotics, that imbalance usually starts with food.

But our Western culture likes to explore feelings, giving them reasons and stories. We believe that when we discover the reason for a feeling, and then get it all worked out, the emotion will dissipate. Personally, I accept both models. I believe that feelings are definitely created by the extreme energies we subject our bodies to—whether that's food or an extreme situation. So it's important to respect that feelings can come from deep cellular memories and old vibrational events as well as last night's dinner.

Sugar and alcohol make for euphoria followed by depression and self-pity. Caffeine makes you bitchy, fearful, and defensive. Meat can cause aggressive feelings, while baked flour leads to irritability. While emotions are natural and necessary, they don't need to regularly take over our lives and wreck our ability to function in the world. As you eat macrobiotically, you will find that, although you feel your emotions more acutely (because you have less sludge), they lessen in intensity. Drama queens become a little boring. Tantrums slip away. Depressed victims find their spines.

When the body is fed macrobiotically, the organs heal themselves. As this occurs, our emotions stabilize and the unecessary ones simply disappear. After becoming macrobiotic, I actually began to feel good most of the time. But because my personality had been built upon a solid foundation of self-pity driven by a dysfunctional childhood and *way* too much sugar for most of my life, I actually had to work for a while in order to accept this happy feeling as my new default mode. So if you need to work out your inner demons with some professional help, go for it. A good counselor or hypnotherapist is a godsend in helping to release old vibrational patterns from your mind and body. Fueled by macrobiotic foods, you will be able to easily let go of old emotional sludge over time. So yell and scream, cry like a baby, and confront that abuser. Let the energy move.

SEX

The furthest thing from "casual," sex is the merging of two energy systems. What quality of energy are you merging with? And considering that everything eventually becomes its opposite, who are you becoming by merging with him or her? Is there room in your relationship to acknowledge the Infinite Universe that brings you together?

When a relationship is toxic, sex can strengthen the abusive bond between two people. When a relationship is healthy, it doubles the healing power of the individuals. Sex can be used to erase resentments or to wield power. How is sex working for you? Later sections in this chapter go into detail about the yin and yang of sex, the foods that affect it, and how macrobiotic eating can serve your sex life.

EXERCISE

Do you exercise regularly? Do you enjoy it?

Extreme foods produce extreme energy and sometimes an urgent need to discharge that energy through exercise. As you eat macrobiotic food, you will experience lots of energy, but not necessarily the same physical urge to push it out just for the sake of pushing it out. With less sludge, it takes less activity to move your energy around. A brisk walk or a vigorous yoga class may suffice, whereas only an hour on the StairMaster would have done the trick before.

In the past, people got lots of exercise. From farming to housecleaning to hauling babies around, women were active from morning till night. But these days, many of us lead relatively sedentary lifestyles. This intertia, coupled with extreme foods, creates the need for gyms where we can "work out" all the excess energy. Heroically, we try to balance our whole sludgy day in less than an hour at the gym, so we push ourselves really hard. But women working farms two hundred years ago never thought, "Boy, if I drag this rake a little faster, I can burn one hundred forty calories in an hour!" Activity was a way of life, and every move was deeply connected to their survival, and the survival of their families. So find activities that you enjoy and feel have purpose for you.

Although regular exercise that breaks a sweat is ideal, also keep your sights on staying active within your life, and cooking is a good place to start. Macrobiotic cooking is quite physical—it requires lifting and pressing and pouring and stirring. Plus, it takes a while. The more active you are in your cooking, the more active you will be in your life.

RELATIONSHIPS

How much energy do you devote to other people? What is the quality of that energy? Supportive and productive? Negative and resentful?

When your chakras start to interact with someone else's, a relationship is born. But we have all sorts of different kinds of relationships; some are casual, some purely professional, while others are lifelong family ties. As you release your sludge, both physical and emotional, you will begin to get real clarity about your relationships. Are you giving, giving, giving, feeling depleted after seeing a friend? Maybe you need to give a little less in order to maintain your balance. Perhaps your sludge armor protected you energetically from certain individuals who now overwhelm you. How do you let your energy move in relationships? Are you honest about your opinions and needs? Or do you hold your truth back, hoping to keep everyone comfortable and happy? Do you talk behind people's backs? Do you depend too much on others, creating resentment in them?

Because we are being created by yin and yang forces every second of every day, our primary relationship is with the Infinite Universe itself. If yin and yang were to simply give up, we'd disappear in a second. So, in order for our human relationships to stay clear, healthy, and growth producing, we need to continually get nourishment from the universe. This comes through good food and spiritual pursuits. When we lean on the universe more than we lean on individuals, our relationships become opportunities for love, laughter, and transformation.

As you continue to eat macrobiotically, you will automatically strengthen your connection to the universe, which will automatically clean up your connections with people. Your intuition will begin to tell you what feels right and what's too much. Healthy relationships begin to develop, and strong bonds of unconditional love emerge.

CREATIVITY

Do you have creative outlets? I believe that creativity is simply the Infinite Universe working through us. Constantly creating (and uncreating) it demands that, as we become healthier and tuned in to its pulse, we carry on the creativity. This doesn't mean you have to take a macramé class, but whatever you are interested in—whatever turns you on—should be pursued. If you're not sure where to start, begin with your cooking; allow yourself to make tiny, daring choices in the kitchen—cut the carrot a funky new way or go with your intuition on a garnish. By following your inner visions as they come, you will open up that creative vortex we all have inside.

When the liver is blocked and stuffy, creativity is thwarted. A stuffy liver makes for impatience and irritable energy. Foods that irritate the liver include too much animal food, baked flour products, heavy and oily foods, and too much salt. The liver loves upward-growing, green foods. When the liver is clean and clear to perform its detoxifying functions, patience and creativity are natural by-products. So if I am struggling with writer's block, I simply avoid the extremes and chew very well, granting the Infinite Universe room to move through me again.

And remember, we don't decide what we will create, just as we don't decide (yet, thank God) the genetic assemblage of our children. It's about being healthy, relaxing, and letting the Infinite Universe give you one instruction at a time.

EXPRESSION

Are you honest? Do you ask to have your needs met? Do you stand up for what you believe in? Are you listened to at work and in your home?

One of the best ways to stay healthy is to continually tell the truth about what you feel and perceive. Whether it's to your journal, your partner, or your therapist, your reality needs to be expressed in order to keep your energy moving and your life healthy. Sometimes it's not appropriate to say everything you feel straight to the offending party, but make sure it comes out in writing or to another person, so the energy moves and you can figure out what to do about the situation. Ask the universe for strength and the ability to be honest and you will always have integrity—another word for "wholeness."

WORK/DREAM

What do you do to bring home the barley? Do you feel it has meaning—to you personally and in the world? Do you enjoy it? Do you *care?* It is a lot easier and more pleasant to commit energy to something you care about. Over time, if you work at a job you have no deep connection to, parts of your being begin to stagnate, go to sleep, die. Conversely, if you are passionate and useful, you get more and more energy to channel because you are considered, in the universe's eyes, responsible and efficient within the economy. You are being given the business because you have proven you can handle it.

I encourage you to find out what your passions are and commit at *least* one hour a week to exploring those passions. Set a timer and write for an hour. Draw. Run a couple of miles and fantasize about doing a marathon. Go hear a political candidate speak and get your juices going about that. Buy a camera. Respond to a personal ad. Just let that secret energy move.

Some of us claim not to know what our dreams are, but here are some tips: what did you dream about being as a kid? There's usually a lot of power stuck in that "silly" dream left behind in childhood. So you wanted to be a ballerina, and now you're approaching thirty with a midriff that Balanchine would laugh at? So what! Taking a dance class now will activate and mobilize that core energy, and *that* is all that matters. It is that core energy that heals your body, connects you with God, and shows you the next right step on your personal path. By eating macrobiotically, you will become more tuned in to your dream and have the good health to pursue it.

George Ohsawa believed that the only reason to recover one's health was to passionately pursue one's dream—that's what life's all about. Likewise, if you don't pay attention to your dream, it will be difficult to maintain your health and balance. So look carefully under the rocks of your consciousness that say, "I'll never do that" or "That's crazy," and just dare to dream—for a second—and you'll find the pirate's gold of your deepest self. Especially if you're in a nowheresville job, it is crucial to let trickle that tributary of connectedness to your true energy, your authentic self, in order to let it surge like the river that it is. By the time it is a river, the crummy job will just evaporate. And you will feel like a million bucks. I know this might sound scary. It is scary to begin living life from your core. It is scary to be passionate. It's scary to be totally free. But Madonna did it.

SPIRITUAL PURSUITS

Do you ever contemplate the bigger picture of the universe? Do you pray, meditate, or have a religious practice? When we contemplate God, we open up to and align with higher, smoother vibrations, automatically discharging sludge.

Whole grains feed your spirit, your soul, your essence. As you eat macrobiotically, you will experience your own wholeness—body, mind, and spirit as one. This easy integration lends itself beautifully to whatever spiritual path you choose to follow. You may find that concepts or practices that felt hollow before make perfect sense now. When I am in the presence of other people—macro or not—who are committed to aligning with the Infinite Universe, no matter what they call it, their faith and energy buoy me automatically. The wholeness I am granted by eating whole grains responds automatically to readings, rituals, and people who discuss the concept of God. Let yourself be nourished with the vibrational foods of love and service, and you will find that your whole-grain wholeness is a great gift to whatever spiritual community you belong to.

warning: getting too yang
on the macro diet

Athletes run the risk of becoming obsessed. Doctors run the risk of thinking they're god. Macrobiotic people run the risk of getting too yang. This is a phenomenon I have witnessed many times within the macrobiotic community. You see, most people walking around are a combination of extreme yin and extreme yang, striking what is basically a dodgy balance. But the macrobiotic diet takes out the extremes so that you're "playing tennis on a much smaller court." On this small court, it is much easier to overdo contraction—within the normal macrobiotic ingredients—than to overdo expansion. Because one pinch of salt can contract you mightily, but one pinch of rice syrup will not deliver the similar amount of expansion. We are no longer playing with the wide extremes of wheat and sugar. Everything has been scaled down a few sizes. And the things to be aware of now—on this new tennis court—are salt and other forms of yang force.

One of the biggest and most insidious problems with becoming too yang is that really yang people cannot recognize their yangness. If anything, they think that they're too yin and—like a strict parent—try to yangize themselves even more. Big yang attracts small yang. I have done this, and it is a strange phenomenon. Because both yin and yang are always present, it can be very tricky diagnosing yourself, but—when in doubt—assume that you're too yang, make the suggested adjustments, and see how you feel.

SIGNS OF BECOMING TOO YANG

The following are signs that you may be becoming too yang:

Extreme weight loss
Lack of outward, expressive energy
Feeling stuck
Feeling tightly wound, unable to relax
Salty taste in mouth

Strong, compulsive cravings for sweets, oil, more salt, or big volumes of
  food
Hard, compact bowel movements
General irritability
Retaining water
Stiffness, especially in back, shoulders, or neck
Headaches at the back of the head
Dark circles under the eyes
Resenting others, thinking they're too loose, chaotic, out of control
Feelings of superiority—not jiving with the rest of the world
Inability or unwillingness to self-reflect on one's own behavior
Having difficulty sitting still
Coldness in extremities

Saltiness can come from these sources: miso, shoyu, umeboshi plums and vinegar, sea vegetables, sea salt, condiments, and pickles. Yangness also comes from baked food (especially baked flour), animal food, long-cooked foods and leftovers, pressure cooking, and eating too much grain. Lack of freshness, and lack of vegetables (especially green ones) or lack of variety can also cause extreme yangness. It is the daily challenge of macro people to keep their conditions loose, light, and outward.

WAYS TO REDUCE EXCESS YANG

After all you have learned, it may seem that the simplest way to reduce excess yang is to add excess yin! Won't they simply balance each other out? Yes, by introducing strong yin, you will probably feel a reduction in the symptoms, but the deep, underlying contraction taking place inside of you will not be released until the strong yang factors are reduced. So make sure you reduce the contraction as much as increasing expansion.

FOOD SUGGESTIONS

Reduce salt to almost nil for a while.

Drink shiitake tea (desalinates the body, p. 182).

Minimize or avoid baked flour products.

Keep fish consumption to a couple of times a week, maximum.

Skip grain at some meals.

Avoid baking and pressure-cooking until you feel better.

Emphasize lighter cooking styles, like nabe-style vegetables.

Eat fresh salads.

Eat a little fruit every day or every other day.

Cook with sweets like rice syrup, barley malt, and amasake.

Drink some warm apple juice a couple of times a week.

Drink warm carrot juice a couple of times a week (yes, warm).

Sip a beer.

LIFESTYLE SUGGESTIONS

Take a hot bath (desalinates the body).

Do relaxation techniques you know.

Get some fresh air.

Get light exercise, preferably outdoors.

Walk barefoot on green, dewy grass.

Surround yourself with warm, loving companionship—people with whom you relax.

Hang out with safe, noncompetitive women (good-quality yin).

Write in your journal to get stuff off your chest—release resentments and fears to the Infinite Universe.

Laugh and be goofy with kids.

Dance.

Sing or hum.

Read spiritual literature or join in spiritual pursuits.

Begin to cultivate the belief that simply "being" is not only enough but a great gift to yourself and everyone around you.

the yin and yang of love

At twenty-seven years old, I left the hyped-up atmosphere of New York City and moved into a macrobiotic community. I was looking forward to a mellow crowd. "Perhaps they will be peaceniks," I mused, "or poets or gardeners." I pictured bearded guys named Lake with patchouli-soaked guitars released from the more mundane conflicts of Saturday-night fistfights. And—looking back now—I assumed that the lack of testosterone-laden red meat in their diets would make them not only warm and fuzzy, but a little . . . *sexually* tame as well.

Nuh-uh. These were very horny guys. Without guitars. Don't get me wrong: there was no wild copulation in the hallways, no tahini-slathered orgies; there was nothing downright weird or extraordinary. It was simply that, whereas in the regular world it is a given that a man's sex drive begins its descent after thirty-five and is on a slow curve down forever more, these guys seemed to be going at it happily into their sixties and seventies, with genuine vigor. At first I assumed it was just talk, but then I noticed that they were unusually strong and sparky in every other way; their faces were animated, their interests wide and varied; they got up with the sun and worked happily all day long. It began to make sense that they would still be able to express their sexual energy with gusto, too. But they didn't look like classic sex machines—no leather jackets, greasy hair, or blown-up biceps. In fact, most of these men were rail thin and ridiculously flexible. What was going on?

Although the women didn't seem quite as overtly randy, they were wonderfully at ease with their sexuality, too; sex as a subject was discussed with a refreshing nonchalance, since it was viewed as a natural and pleasurable part of a healthy person's life. Just as we breathe, perspire, urinate, and poop, so must we release sexual energy and fluids. And without sludge building up around their reproductive organs, these macrobiotic people were free to experience this energy in a normal, unimpeded way. Finally, without physical blockage around their sexuality, there was no mental or emotional blockage on the subject, either. Years of shame and negativity I had carried within me, programming I received from my childhood and our culture, began to fall away.

And then I fell in love. When it came time for me to explore this energy with a macrobiotic man, the magnetic pull I felt to him was so intense it almost hurt. Before we were prepared to be honest about our feelings, our friends and classmates named it for us: "You guys are in love," they said. "Just admit it." But our wary egos had not yet caught up with our souls. Without ever touching each other, our chakras had opened up an energy circuit between us, aching to achieve that unity that lies behind duality. More sensitive friends even said that they could see this lovely energy between us, that when we were together, each one of us changed, softened, and opened in the most amazing way. This transference and balancing of forces was healing, causing each of us to look and feel like a million bucks. And when the physical connection finally took place, our bodies, much more spark than sludge, caused a local power outage. Just kidding. But it was good.

So let's look at how all this works through a macrobiotic lens. Remember that we are each—as individuals—the amazing meeting of yin and yang energies. Yang enters at the head and yin at the perineum, and they collide to create spirals called chakras. From the chakras, energy pours along the meridians, into the palms of the hands, soles of the feet, and farther downriver at the tips of the fingers and toes. This is the energy that we bring to our sexual experiences.

Men are governed by the yang energy entering from the cosmos, and women are governed by the yin energy coming from the earth. This difference in governing force is easily recognized on the physical level.

In women, yin force issuing from the earth creates upward, hollow, expanded phenomena as it creates the vagina, the uterus, and the fallopian tubes, which reach out to the estrogen-producing ovaries. All this yin energy actually results in a yang product, the ovum. The center of gravity of this female body is lower, closer to the earth, which is its source. As we watch the yin energy moving upward, it creates the expanded, fatty tissue of breasts, as well as an overall softness of the body. Fat is more yin and muscle is more yang. The woman also has softer, lighter body hair.

Meanwhile, the man is governed by a force coming in at the top of his head. The first sexual organ of a man is his mind. Images especially serve as sparks to his sexual ignition. His center of gravity is more upward in the body, at the chest, and the overall hardness and density of his muscles show us the contracting, yang force that governs him. As we move down the body, it is getting slimmer, like the spiral that is creating it, and finally the spiral contracts to a point at the tip of the penis. This is the most sensitive and highly charged point of a man's body. All this yang energy results in a more yin substance, semen.

As we imagine the bodies side by side, we realize that the genders are truly complementary opposites; it's as if the inifinite universe made one model of human and then stretched some of us in one direction while the other half got pulled the other way. We both have nipples, but those of a man are basically functionless. We both have shoulders, but those of a woman are nothing like as strong as a man's. The long, hollow vagina is the perfect complementary opposite to the long, erect penis, and the testes and ovaries are both seed-producing machines—it's just that one set is stored in a sac outside the boy while its cousins are placed apart daintily, like teacups, inside the girl. Hormonally, we have lots of the same ingredients, but women have the market on estrogen (more yin), while guys hold stock in testosterone (more yang).

With all these complementary antagonistic opposites, it's no wonder country music thrives. Let's take a look at what happens when yin and yang get close and the energy builds. Imagine you are standing in a low-lit room waiting for your lover. He is either (a) the current love of your life, or (b) a major television or motion-picture hottie. Pick one. As the soon-to-be lovers come together, the electricity in the air is real. Your spiralic chakras, governed by opposite forces, attract each other fiercely. You both behave in order to entice each other. You intuitively move in ways to excite him visually; he responds by whispering compliments in your ear, warm and slow, which causes your chakras to relax and open up more. Sexy thoughts fly through the air, literally charging the atmosphere. At the perfect moment, you touch his leg, which sends the signal that the stakes have been raised; the tension is reaching a new level and heartbeats have increased, breathing is heavy and the spirals are running the show.

For yin and yang to unite, there must be a sustained building of tension before an explosive union occurs. So you both continue, using all your intuitive tricks. Saliva is highly charged energetically, and when his yang-charged saliva meets your yin-charged saliva, the passionate kissing that takes place at one end of the spine sends fireworks down to the other. If he hasn't got one already, your man gets an erection and you secretly secrete vaginal fluids, also highly charged energetically and the polar opposite of semen. This is where the radio transmitters come into it—heaven's force is literally pouring down his spine, beginning at the brain (where men are initially sexually stimulated—he's thinking about how good you look) and moving down, opening all his chakras, but concentrating itself at the other end of the spine, where his reproductive organs reside. This energy also flows out along invisible energy pathways called meridians, in his arms and legs, causing secondary chakras in the palms of the hands and soles of the feet to open. He feels a desperate need to touch you all over to let yang meet yin.

Meanwhile, as our heroine, you are receiving the opposite charge in the form of yin force, causing your vagina to open and lubricate, your labia and clitoris to become engorged with blood. That whole area of your body feels warm and is beginning to pulsate as blood charges your pelvic area and responds energetically to the action taking place in his pelvic area. The expansive, yin energy issuing from the earth continues up your spine, releasing itself in a more diffuse way as love courses through your heart, voice, and mind. You feel connected to this man more deeply than words could ever express. It goes beyond the mind, beyond the body, as yang meets yin. You fool around a little more, and eventually, with penetration, the vibrational exchange intensifies. Add a little friction, and your identities melt into each other.

If the radio transmitters are sludgy and unable to conduct this force easily, the sexual spark between the two of you is dull and the depth of connection reduced. With clean radio transmitters, the energy flows smoothly, allowing blood to go to all the right places, the sexual tension to build naturally, gathering at the chakras, causing the fingers and toes to curl, the face to scrunch up as the friction increases and increases and . . . kaboom! One or both of you climax. The orgasmic release is unimpeded, ecstatic, and warmly satisfying, causing all the pent-up energy to flow deliciously back to the rest of the body, newly balanced by your lover's opposite energy.

This feeling is the afterglow of sex, where all the previous tension has been released and each partner feels full and connected to the other. On an energetic level, the man has deposited heaven's force (yang) into you through his penis, and you have released earth's force (yin) into him from your heart. Together, the circuit of energy that is created is bigger than the sum of its parts and can feel like the universe re-creating itself, which, when a new life begins, is exactly what is happening.

So that's perfect, hot sex. But is that what always happens? These days, all sorts of sexual issues are coming out into the light of day: erectile dysfunction, frigidity, infertility, lack of interest between couples after only a short time together. What is going on?

Unless you just picked up this book and went straight to the sex section, you should understand by now some of the energy reasons that our sexuality can get into trouble. If yin and yang seek union through men and women, and men are governed by yang and women are governed by yin, then it makes sense for women to try to stay a little yin while men stay a little yang in order to maintain an active energy charge between them. So, our problems begin when either member of the couple starts getting out of balance in some way.

to my gay and bi readers

Although this writing comes from my hetero perspective, gay relationships follow the principles of yin and yang in their own way; in most same-sex couples, there is one member who is more yang and one who is more yin. And although nothing is black and white, look at yourself and your partner to decide: is one of you more extroverted and the other more introverted? Who is more traditionally "masculine" and who is more "feminine"? Which one of you is more emotionally sensitive? Try to figure out who is more governed by yang and who is more governed by yin—and there should be strong differences between you on a few levels or there would be no attraction.

With respect to food, by eliminating the extremes from your diet and eating whole foods, your relationship will automatically become more peaceful and harmonious. But you may also experiment with one partner eating a little more yang food while the other consciously chooses more yin food. By doing this, you are manipulating the energy charge between you. Notice if the polarity between you gets stronger or more dynamic. Then have some real fun by trading roles—and diets—and see what happens! What works best for your compatibility? Your sex life? Considering that you are both the same gender, you can actually experiment with more flexibilty than a straight couple can.

WHEN A WOMAN GETS TOO YANG

It's easy these days for women to get too much yang energy. Eating animal foods three times a day, along with baked flour products and lots of salt, multiplied by a stressful world and an equally stressful career, it's amazing these days that women have any sex at all.

But we do. Because animal products, which include testosterone, will grant us the male side of our sexual coin, which is fun, a little aggressive, and concentrated on our little counterpart to the penis, the clitoris. This type of sex tends to be all about orgasm, as if that were the be-all and end-all of female sexuality. Bedding someone feels more like a business deal: "I'll give you your orgasm if you give me mine." And there can be lots of pressure, which is also a yang quality, to both perform and to validate the man's performance correctly by having the requisite orgasm.

But, unfortunately, the saturated fat found in animal foods will impede blood flow to the pelvic area, including the clitoris, and can decrease energetic conductivity along the walls of the vagina. Although there are no nerve endings past the first inch of the vagina, this is the locus of most friction created with her energetically opposite partner and therefore the place of most vibrational exchange. It is where the partners literally merge. If the walls of the vagina are dulled by the buildup of saturated fat, insufficient lubrication occurs, and the woman cannot receive her partner's vibrations as nature intends, impeding their sense of union. Her female receptivity, which characterizes her sexuality, is thwarted. The picture here is not so much about energy, receptivity, or union but about sensory pleasure and the ego.

With the continued buildup of saturated fat can come complications such as blocked fallopian tubes, cysts, and fibroid tumors. Cancer of the reproductive organs has been linked to the consumption of saturated fat. Frequent white or cloudy vaginal discharge is actually sludge and should basically cease with good macrobiotic practice.

WHEN A MAN GETS TOO YIN

Men are eating foods these days that were simply not available to them a hundred years ago. Ice cream, soda, chocolate, iced beverages, artificial sweeteners, tropical fruits, and prescription medication have all become regular parts of the average guy's fare. And let's not forget beer or other forms of alcohol, which are also very yin. These substances are so yin that they weaken the yang spiral entering the man.

But let's see what happens up close in terms of sexual vigor: in order to function sexually, a guy's most pressing issue, physically, is the ability to maintain an erection. And strong erections are the result of both good-quality yang and good-quality yin. The yang component is the blood itself, highly charged, hot, moving downward in the body. The yin part goes like this: during arousal, nerves are stimulated that cause the two large spongy masses of muscle that comprise the sides of the penis to relax, thereby drawing in extra blood. Very soon, this extra blood produces a hardness (yang) that helps to clamp down on veins that normally bring blood out of the penis. When too much yin energy is taken in by the man, the initial nerve response that causes the erection to occur becomes weak or deadened. Too much yin energy causes the veins that hold blood in the penis to become weak, never allowing the clamping to occur. That's a problem. And when a man detects that he has any issue with achieving or maintaining an erection, a self-consciousness occurs that triggers fear and withdrawal.

The coldness inherent in ice cream, soda pop, and other icy beverages also inhibits the heat of sexuality, both male and female. When the body is forced to use its energy to heat up the stuff going inside of it, chakra power is reduced and the sexual dynamic suffers.

WHEN WOMEN BECOME TOO YIN

Yes, we can overdo our own natural energy. When a woman lives on salads, fruit, diet soda, frozen yogurt, and chocolate, she becomes too expanded. Her blood becomes weak and demineralized. Eventually, she may become sort of an invisible, codependent ghost, sucking out of other people the life force she lacks to survive.

Her natural attribute of sensitivity goes out of whack and she is hypersensitive, crying without provocation. A self-centeredness can come about, which is the exact opposite of the yang pigheadedness we can sometimes see in men; she is plagued by low self-esteem, needs constant reassurance, and leans on her friends and family with her bottomless pit of needs. It's as if the flower had opened and opened and opened until its petals started shooting off the stem. Hysterical freakouts may occur. She can be scattered, compulsively talky, and easily fatigued, as the energy just keeps on spiraling out.

Eventually, because there is so little contraction compared with expansion, her core feels empty, and this is the black hole that can never be filled by anyone or any cake or any Prada shoe. Sexually speaking, this woman may display excessive body shame, an inability to relax into sex, and even "frigidity" because her core has become so expanded and cold. She lacks the good-quality yang of downward-moving blood and the sexual heat that goes with it. Too much yin can also inhibit her ability to hold the energy in her uterus to carry a baby to term. This is yin gone bad. Worst-case scenarios include chronic depression and suicide.

menstruation

As we all know, women go through a complete hormonal cycle roughly every twenty-eight days. And like every natural cycle, it is a complete trip from yin to yang and back again. The menstrual cycle consists of two phases. First, during the time between menstruation and ovulation the uterus is repairing its lining, or endometrium. The body is concentrating its energy toward this effort and toward the follicle maturing in the ovary. This phase is more yang. Second, during ovulation when the ovum is released, extreme yang becomes yin, and we enter phase two. If the ovum is not fertilized, the body becomes more yin, prepares to shed the endometrium, and phase two concludes with the hormonal signal to release. If however, the ovum is fertilized, the body goes on a completely different journey of pregnancy (which is very yang), but is too complicated to cover here in detail.

So why do you crave chocolate right before your period? Let's think of it this way: in summer, you crave foods that help you to align with the season—fruits, salads, and other good stuff that cause expansion. In winter, you gravitate toward foods that contract you. Using that same intuition, women naturally crave expanders like sugar, chocolate, and sometimes alcohol right before their periods, which is the time of greatest expansion. So you're doing fine already. However, if you are also eating lots of meat, chicken, eggs, salt, dairy, and baked flour (all very yang), you are inviting in as much (if not more) contraction than expansion. Eating these foods during phase two of your cycle is like eating ice cream in winter. It goes against the tide. Too much yang energy in the body can lead to cramping, backaches, headaches, or even more serious menstrual complications. So, if you are feeling the onset of PMS, do yourself a favor and go easy on the yang foods:

- Reduce or eliminate fish or any other animal food.
- Reduce salt intake—go easy on seasonings, pickles, and condiments.
- Reduce or eliminate all bread and baked flour products—you'll thank me.
- Avoid white sugar. But go for sweets like rice syrup, barley malt, or even maple syrup.
- Emphasize leafy greens and lighter cooking styles.
- Feel free to reduce whole grains, emphasizing vegetables and grain products.
- Go for lighter grain dishes like bulghur wheat, couscous, and noodles.
- Have some fruit.
- If you're in good health, relax with a Rice Dream Chocolate Sundae (see p. 119).
- If you're in good health (and not a recovering alcoholic), have a beer or some sake.

Staying yin by eating good-quality macrobiotic foods can make your period a comfortable, even joyous expression of your alignment with nature. For lessening menstrual cramps, see Daikon Drink (p. 183).

WHEN MEN BECOME TOO YANG

When a guy eats meat, eggs, and cheese all the time, saturated fat builds up in his arteries. We all know the dangers of saturated fat with respect to the heart, but saturated fat goes just as readily to the arteries entering the penis. When there is blockage along these little highways, only a trickle of traffic can get through, and that's not enough to create an erection.

Saturated fat, in conjunction with strong yin foods, can result in an enlarged prostate. It also creates an energetic dullness throughout the whole body that reduces overall sensitivity. Meat's strong yang energy drives the focus down into the penis so completely that the other chakras—heart, voice, mind—remain tight and closed. This means that lots of guys totally miss the vibrational exchange that is sex. Too much animal food also supports a self-centeredness that blocks the natural generosity and connectedness that sexual exchange brings out in people. Meat contains testosterone, and men who eat lots and lots of meat build up lots and lots of testosterone. This excess of male sexual hormones can create unnatural urgency around the sexual act, resulting in premature ejaculation.

The worst-case scenario is that men can become so yang that they themselves revert to animal behavior. Yes, a sweaty quickie can be fun, but aggressive, violent behavior in the bedroom is no longer human.

Of course, most people dabble in both extremes of the energy spectrum; meat-eating men may drink alcohol, making them remorseful, depressed thugs, and chocoholic women may eat a chicken breast daily, making them hysterical, needy control freaks. Yikes.

WE'RE BOTH BOTH

Because yin and yang are always together, each gender has two types of sexual expression. However, women are naturally governed by the force that causes us to be open, sensitive, and receptive. We are physically designed to literally "receive" our partners. Sometimes yin energy is described as "passive," and I don't like that, because it sounds like rolling over and playing dead. Yin energy actively receives, lets in, absorbs. It is as active as yang energy, but in the other direction. Energetically, this is our dominant mode.

The yang side of our sexuality is to achieve an orgasm, whether it's via the clitoris, the vagina, or a combination of both. But this our secondary mode. As any woman knows, our sexual energy changes throughout the month, and throughout a lifetime. Yes, sometimes we crave an orgasm, but there are other times when we feel very sexual, without caring about an orgasm at all. There are even times of the month when—hormonally—it goes against the grain to attempt to have an orgasm, and yet intercourse and connection with a partner feel absolutely sublime. Women, being governed by yin, are governed by variability. What excited you in your twenties may seem totally boring to you now, and your current deep, loving, satisfying contact with your partner would have seemed like dullsville to your inner seventeen-year-old. Sometimes we want to be on top, and sometimes we want to be spooned. Sometimes we want to be taken by surprise.

What I see taking place in our culture is that we are acknowledging only the yang side of our sexuality. Orgasm, orgasm, orgasm. One-night stands. Women becoming as tough and as heartless as we used to complain men were. I trust that this is a combination of the pendulum swinging to its opposite direction after millennia of sexual repression and an increase in animal food consumption in the last fifty years. What has occurred is very natural, considering the pendulum of patriarchy needed to start swinging in our favor. But politics will never transcend the order of the universe, and as long as we are biologically female, we are governed by yin.

Now, ladies, I am not trying to take away our orgasm. Orgasms are wonderful and natural, and a more balanced, grain-based diet will allow you to have fantastic ones. But it is important to know that, because we are governed by earth's force, we have more in our sexual pleasure chest than an orgasm, and the more we eat and make love with receptivity in mind, the better everything becomes. A grain-based diet that minimizes saturated fat allows the vagina—the place where yin and yang rendezvous—to be highly charged and sensitive to the energy exchange. This same lack of saturated fat allows your entire body, so alive, so sensitive, so (as Freud termed it) "polymorphously perverse" to be a five-foot-six-inch sex organ.

HEALTHY YIN ENERGY—A WOMAN'S ADVANTAGE

Poor guys. Let them be the ones to focus exclusively on "coming." We've already arrived! Their spirals demand a buildup of energy that "comes" to a point of no return in order to be satisfied. And because we receive heaven's force, too, we also enjoy that pleasurable capability, but our dominant, expansive spiral allows us to release energetically all over the place, our female, earthy love allows us to connect us not just sexually but spiritually with our partners.

Healthy yin is the force issuing up and out into the universe. Currently believed to be on expand mode, the universe courses up and through a woman, pulling both partners toward their primary connection with the larger whole. No wonder we got burned as witches. Until the universe starts to contract again (which won't be for a long while), women are the stronger lightning rods of the invisible world. Men ground us, protect us, and dominate the material concerns of the planet, but we bring the universe to the table. When a woman gets in touch with this *huge* energy coursing through her, an orgasm looks nice, but sort of provincial. You are a healer in the bedroom: a witch, a saint, a goddess. Relax, receive, and let love course through you.

Healthy yin energy is also the stuff of relationships. Without it, we would all be playing vigorous soccer for eternity. And the more a woman honors her yin strength, an invisible force that acts like an intoxicating magnetic perfume, the more she can attract and sustain beautiful relationships. Our culture teaches us to force and control and guarantee our fates, as well as our mates—but that is a male (yang) model based on contraction, exactly the opposite of the energy that governs us. Forgiveness, softness, and an intuitive connection to the Infinite Universe are the secret weapons, as it were, in our relationships. By relaxing and letting good-quality yin energy pour through, we automatically attract the yang force of men because they need it to balance themselves out, just as we need them.

Because our spiral is about expansion, we respond differently to matters sexual: women usually need some sort of emotional wooing before opening up sexually. We need to feel supported and loved, secure in the relationship. Love, support, and security make up the petri dish for more expansion—the opening of our sexual "flower." Even if women can become aroused without these ele-ments, enjoying the thrill of a one-night stand now and again, it is difficult for us to sustain a sexual relationship on a casual basis because the very act of inter-course (an expansive act for us) opens our emotionally and bonds us to our part-ner in a very deep way. This is the basis for our "Fatal Attraction" cliché of the obsessive female stalker, bonded to a man way beyond his comprehension from a single act of intercourse. To him, he has simply acted casually, like a bee land-ing on a flower, and can move on easily. But she has literally been entered—physically, emotionally, and energetically. Governed by the receptive yin spiral of earth's force, she has "received" him and it is difficult to let him go. On a phys-iological level, arousal causes her to dose herself with oxytocin, which is a strong bonding hormone. On a mental level, because her energy field has been entered by him, her clear judgment literally becomes obscured by his energy. It is quite easy for women to "lose" themselves to a sexual relationship. One good reason not to sleep with someone too fast.

And this is the way nature intends it. It shouldn't be that easy for a woman to "get over" people she has received and loved. Imagine if it were energetically easy for women to "let go of" or "get over" their children—we wouldn't have a human race! Babies just plopped down on highways when Mom gets bored or forgetful is not in nature's overall plan. It's yin force that receives and bonds, and it's yang force that creates boundaries. Both are vital to the happy functioning of both genders. But next time you feel like a total idiot because you still think about him six months after the breakup and he's moved on to the next "flower," remember that you are governed by the energy that unites and bonds human be-ings with love and that's nothing to be ashamed of. He has the uniting energy, too, but it's just easier for him to take action sooner, because he is governed by yang. That's why you have girlfriends to cry to; they, governed by yin, can "receive" you as you grieve the loss and remind you that there are other fish in the sea.

Men have yin and yang sides of their sexuality, too. Because they are gov-erned by yang, an orgasm is usually a necessary component in sexual satisfaction. And the male buildup of energy toward an explosive orgasm brings a nice hot dynamic to the bedroom. Male sexual hormones bring protectiveness, playful aggression, and conquest to the table. Yang energy allows men to cut off from intimacy more easily than women do, and this ability to shut down allows them to experience sex more casually, if desired. This quality is probably as biologi-cally mandated as our instant bonding, so that his forebears could kill something (without breaking down in tears) in order to feed or protect the family. Because men are governed by yang force, their feelings (more yin) can get pushed down deep inside, having a hard time seeing the light of day. This also makes men (generally) the better breaker-uppers.

But because we are both both, men also want to be cuddled and adored, ex-changing love as much as fluids with their partners. They also secrete the hor-mone oxytocin. That is as natural to them as our enjoying an orgasm.

Luckily, everyone has the capability to experience sex as a mind-blowing, bonding, vibrational meeting of yin and yang *and* feel that incredible love that comes through us as yin and yang reach out to each other *and* have a hell of a good time in our bodies.

EATING FOR A BETTER RELATIONSHIP

One of the most important dimensions of a good relationship is the mainte-nance of attraction, and attraction exists on the energy plane. I quote the French by saying that often we are attracted by a *je ne sais quoi* in our partners. This "I don't know what" is a way of expressing that the thing that draws us is neither visual nor material nor intellectual. It is inexplicable. Pure energy. And it is very exciting. Keeping that energy alive and strong is the job of the individuals in a relationship in order to maintain the sexual magnetism.

This is important not just for a great sex life. It is important because it is this primal spark that unites the partners on other levels, too. If this pull exists be-tween you, it can help you work creatively together as parents or partners real-izing a shared dream. With the magnetism drawing you together, you are more likely to find ways to work through emotional or ideological differences, help-ing each other to grow as friends. With the pull of the spirals strong, a channel opens up for love to flow, whether it is expressed sexually, verbally, or through just a tender kiss.

When we eat the same good-quality food, we are brought to the same ener-getic wavelength. It becomes easier to communicate, to see things from the same angle, to open up vibrationally to each other. But when we are fed from two different sources, we must "get over" the energetic dissonance of the food in order to align. Foods prepared by other people are fine for variety's sake, but between the questionable ingredients and the quality of the cook's energy, we are leaving our bodies, minds, and relationships at the mercy of strangers. And it has become really common these days for couples to eat apart on a regular basis. He brings home his takeout, while she makes her diet microwave dinner. He picks up his lunch at the deli while she goes to the cafeteria at work.

But your relationship is like a plant; it must be fed and cared for. When you cook for your partner, or he cooks for you, your relationship is being nourished. Nourished on a level deeper than talking, therapy, or even sex, for by cooking good-quality food with love, you are literally charging the cells of the body and mind that show up for the marriage counselor's office, or show up in bed. Cooking is downright radical.

Both partners need good-quality food in order to maintain their health. So whole foods respecting nature's yin-to-yang ratio are necessary and will facilitate compatibility. But keeping in mind that women are more yin and men are more yang, we each need to make our own particular choices within macrobiotic quality fare in order to maintain the natural polarity between yin and yang.

It's no accident that girls were made of "sugar and spice" in the old rhyme. Nor that boys were made of "snails and puppy-dog tails." Women can handle more yin foods like sweets, fresh salads, and lighter seasonings. Females tend to do better with more vegetables and less grain. Men tend to go for, and are nourished by, more animal food, more seasoning, and less strong yin. They are generally more attracted to grain than vegetables.

But let's get practical here: you're probably not reading this book together, and he's about as far from a sea vegetable as he is from Mars, so how is it going to all work? If your partner wants nothing to do with this "macro hooey," don't worry. You can't force this stuff on anyone. Just make some things like really yummy, rich, savory fried rice. Or go crazy with a good fish dish. If he is closed off to the idea, do *not,* under any circumstances, utter the word *macrobiotic* to him. Just include a dish here, and a dish there, and let him refuse them if they're not to his liking. You will find that, somewhere along the line, he's picking at the leftover noodles or that the crispy rice treat tray is empty. Food is food, and if it's delicious, he'll forget that it's the "weird fad" you're into. The goal is to continually improve the quality of your life, which will have an impact on the ones around you.

If your partner is really into macrobiotics and he gave you this book for your birthday, don't despair. If the two of you decide to improve your lives through the kitchen, you have made a very powerful choice. Just keep an open mind, be willing to learn, and when it all seems like too much, eat whatever you want.

If you are both interested in macrobiotics, then cook the recipes in this book and continue to study the subject by reading other books, attending cooking classes, and getting to know other people who practice macrobiotics. Women should go a little easier on the salt, condiments, pickles (rinse them well), and grain. Men can enjoy more seitan, burdock, bread, fish, and salty foods, while the ladies hover over the dessert tray. As you desludge together, you will feel that frisky spark you first felt between you lighting up again.

Go bungee jumping, enjoy romantic getaways, or see a marriage counselor if you need to. Do what is right for you to take care of your relationship, for food is not everything. If resentment or jealousy creeps in, the space between you can get used for antagonism; learning how to discharge those feelings with love is crucial. But isn't it nice to know that if each partner cleans the sludge off her or his individual radio transmitter (the spinal column and chakras)—not just emotionally, but physically—the natural energetic attraction between you will stay strong? With clean and shiny radio transmitters, your partnership can become more respectful, intuitive, and even magical than you ever imagined.

LOVE IS . . .

Well, we've talked about sex, so now let's talk about love. I believe . . . that when it comes to romantic relationships, there's the initial attraction that unites two people, and then the love that sustains them. The former seems to me a function of a bunch of different factors but can be interpreted as a pleasing and highly charged collision of yins and yangs between two unique personalities, or auras. The latter, however, is a universal phenomenon that every person can give, receive, and enjoy.

I have heard in macrobiotic classes that love is the one thing that actually transcends yin and yang because love is the Infinite Universe itself. Whoah. So when a human truly loves, he or she opens to the all-embracing, accepting source of all things.

As you desludge and make room inside your body and consciousness for the universe to barrel through, you are opening yourself to both give and receive more love. But not the dramatic, euphoric, or painful love we see in the movies. Those are just distortions of love. Love is—because it transcends duality—actually neutral. It is listening with a truly open mind and heart. It is giving without expecting something in return. It is accepting unconditionally. You have surely experienced it at different moments in your life. Maybe you already have a conscious practice around unconditional love. Or perhaps you've never really considered the concept.

As your body gets stronger by eating macrobiotically and your whole vibe gets lighter, you will automatically give more positive energy to those closest to you, because you *are* positive energy. At the same time, you may find that you naturally begin to love more and more people, as this wonderful energy extends itself through and out of you much farther than it has before. For such a long time, sludge has been holding you back. But now, as you release, relax, and chew your food, don't get freaked out when you become unstoppable.

conclusion: five tips

1. After going whole hog for at least a year, your body and mind will have desludged quite a bit. You will begin to experience freedom. When you are truly free, with a strong compass and a love for yin and yang, you can eat anything you feel drawn to. When you go to an extreme, your body will let you know, and you will have the willingness and wherewithal to come back home to center.

2. Coming back home to center means going back to whole hog. Even if it's only for a meal. Whenever you feel out of sorts—like you're running around madly between yin and yang in every area of your life—just sit yourself down to a balanced meal and chew it extremely well. The chaos should cease.

If you are indulging in extremes and experience physical discomfort or pain, humbly take it as a sign that you are violating the order of the universe, kick out the sludge, and cook for yourself. You know best how to balance your own condition. You may need to go whole hog for an extended period if you are really out of sorts. If it persists, seek out a counselor who may better be able to identify the imbalance that's occurring.

3. Continue to study macrobiotics. I could only touch upon so much in this book. Stay inspired. Cook. Read. Grow. Teach others. This is a lifelong study with lifelong benefits.

4. Relax and be patient. Freedom doesn't come overnight. It pushes through you—in fits and starts—as the Infinite Universe vies for space in your consciousness. Some growth feels comfortable, and some growth cracks through you like thunder as you lose yourself, becoming one with the next exquisite horizon of the infinite.

5. Have fun.

GLOSSARY OF TERMS

Aduki bean: a small, reddish bean grown in both Japan and the United States. Considered to be very good for the kidneys. Also known as azuki or adzuki.

Agar agar: this sea vegetable comes in the form of bars or flakes. It is used for making gelatins and aspics.

Amasake: a sweetener or drink made from fermented sweet rice. Like a macro milk shake.

Arame: a sea vegetable that comes in thin brown strands. It is used like hijiki, as a regular side dish.

Barley, pearl: see Hato Mugi.

Barley malt: a sweetener made from barley. Great in desserts, bean dishes, and tea.

Brown rice: unpolished rice with only its tough outer husk removed.

Brown rice vinegar: a mild vinegar made from fermented brown rice or sweet brown rice.

Burdock: a hardy and tough root vegetable used in stews and various vegetable dishes. Burdock strengthens and purifies the blood. Very good for both genders, but especially strengthening for men.

Couscous: a Moroccan pasta made from wheat, it comes in the form of tiny balls.

Daikon: a long white root vegetable. Used dried or fresh in a variety of vegetable dishes. Especially good for dissolving fat and mucous deposits in the body.

Dried tofu: tofu that has been dried via freezing. Used in a variety of vegetable dishes, dried tofu has less fat than fresh tofu.

Dulse: a reddish purple sea vegetable used in soups, salads, and vegetable dishes. Dulse is high in protein, iron, vitamin A, iodine, and phosphorus.

Flame deflector: a lightweight, round, metal disc perforated with little holes. When placed between a pot and a flame, the deflector allows the heat of the fire to be spread evenly under the pot. This helps to avoid burning during cooking. They can be purchased at health-food stores with cookware sections or at most kitchenware stores. Also known as a flame tamer or flame diffuser.

Gomashio: a condiment made from sesame seeds and sea salt. Normal serving reccommendation is one teaspoon a day. It is especially good for the functioning of the heart.

Grain coffee: a coffee substitute made of roasted grains, beans, and roots. It contains no caffeine. It is considered an occasional beverage.

Green nori flakes: a condiment made from a type of nori different from the one used in sushi rolls. The flakes are rich in iron, calcium, and vitamin A.

Hato Mugi: also known as pearl barley and Job's Tears, this wild grass is cooked as is, with other grains, in soups and stews. It is particularly good at eliminating old animal fats.

Hijiki: a sea vegetable, hijiki comes in dry, black, wiry strands. It should always be rehydrated before cooking. Also known as hiziki.

Hokkaido pumpkin: a type of winter squash very similar to the buttercup and Hubbard varieties. Either deep orange or dark green.

Kanten: a gelled dessert made from agar agar.

Kinpira: a long-cooked vegetable dish traditionally made from carrots and burdock. Other vegetables included in kinpira are lotus root, rutabaga, and green beans. Very strengthening and energizing.

Koji: a grain, usually semi-polished or polished rice, inoculated with bacteria and used to begin the fermentation process in a variety of foods, including miso, amasake, tamari, natto, and sake.

Kombu: a sea vegetable that comes in thick, wide strips. Used in bean dishes, vegetables dishes, condiments, and various home remedies.

Kukicha tea: sometimes called bancha, kukicha tea consists of the twigs and leaves of Japanese twig bushes. High in calcium, kukicha also alkalizes the blood.

Kuzu: a thickener derived from the kudzu plant, which grows wild in the southern United States.

Lotus root: a beige-colored root with hollow chambers inside, lotus root is especially good for the lungs. Used in vegetable dishes and home remedies.

Mirin: cooking wine made from sweet brown rice.

Miso: a protein-rich fermented soybean paste made from ingredients such as soybeans, barley, and brown or white rice. Miso is used in soup stocks and as a seasoning. The most medicinal miso is barley miso aged two years or more. Darker miso aged two years or more does not need to be refrigerated, but younger, lighter misos should be. Miso aids digestion, alkalizes the body, and is considered able to reduce the effects of radiation on the body. There are many different types of miso—rice, chickpea, soybean. Barley miso is used most regularly for daily miso soup.

Mochi: sweet rice steamed and pounded into a cake. Sometimes flavored with raisins, sesame seeds, or other ingredients. It is used as is, in vegetable dishes, or as croutons. A great dish.

Nabe pot: a ceramic pot, usually with a colorfully decorated lid, in which nabe-style vegetables are made.

Nishime: a style of cooking vegetables in which chunks of hearty vegetables are slowly steamed in a heavy, covered pot with kombu sea vegetable at the bottom.

Nori: a sea vegetable pressed into sheets. Untoasted nori is brownish black in color, and toasted or sushi nori is greenish black. Used as a snack, in condiments, and for rolling sushi.

Ohsawa pot: a ceramic pot and lid used for cooking rice or vegetables. The Ohsawa pot is placed in shallow water, inside a stainless-steel pressure cooker, and the whole thing is brought to pressure, as in pressure-cooking.

Pressed salad: thinly sliced vegetables pickled slightly with either sea salt, brown rice vinegar, umeboshi vinegar, or some other pickling agent. The pickling process makes the vegetables more digestible.

Rice syrup: a sweetener made by fermenting brown rice.

Sea salt: salt that is the product of evaporated sea water. The sea salt used in macrobiotic cooking contains no sugar or chemical additives.

Seitan: wheat gluten cooked in a salty broth and then used in stews or as a meat substitute.

Shiitake: usually used in the dried form, shiitake mushrooms are used in soups, stews, and home remedies. They are particularly good at helping the body to dishcharge excess animal fat.

Shiso: also known as a beefsteak leaf, the shiso leaf is used in the pickling of umeboshi plums and gives them their red color.

Shoyu: the Japanese word for soy sauce. Shoyu is used in bean and vegetable dishes and as a seasoning for soups.

Soba: noodles made from buckwheat flour or a combination of buckwheat and whole-wheat flour. Soba can be served in broth, in salads, or with vegetables. In the summer, soba noodles are good chilled.

Somen: very thin white or whole-wheat Japanese noodles. Thinner than soba and other whole-grain noodles, somen are often served during the summer.

Sprouted-wheat bread: a whole-grain bread made from soaked wheat that is sprouted and baked. Sprouted-wheat bread does not contain flour, salt, or oil and is very sweet and moist.

Suribachi: a serrated, ceramic bowl that is sold with a surikogi (see below), it is akin to a mortar and pestle but with the added dimension of the serrated surface, which helps to grind and crush ingredients into fine powders or pastes. A medium-sized set can be found in most good health-food stores. If you are not ready to make this purchase, or simply don't have the time to hand-grind, you can use a handheld food processor to blend ingredients. A large blender or food processor is too big to do the fine crushing needed for gomashio.

Surikogi: a wooden pestle.

Sweet brown rice: a slighty sweet, high-protein, and glutenous form of brown rice. Used in mochi, vinegar, amasake, and other foods.

Tahini: a seed butter made from grinding sesame seeds until smooth and creamy.

Takuan: daikon pickled in sea salt and rice bran.

Tekka: a strong condiment made from miso, sesame oil, burdock, lotus root, carrot, and ginger. Cooked for several hours, it is rich in iron and is usually store-bought as opposed to made at home.

Tempeh: an Indonesian food made from split soybeans and water and is a beneficial bacterial starter. High in protein and, if unpasteurized, also high in vitamin B_{12}.

Tempura: vegetables or seafood battered and deep-fried in unrefined oil.

Tofu: bean curd, made from soybeans and nigari, a natural coagulant. Used in soups, vegetable dishes, and dressings.

Udon: Japanese noodles made from wheat, whole wheat, or whole wheat and unbleached white flour.

Umeboshi: salty, pickled plums. Umeboshi plums alkalize the blood and stimulate salivation and appetite. They are used as pickles, in condiments, cooking grain, and in many home remedies. Umeboshi paste is not as medicinal but is also used as a seasoning.

Umeboshi vinegar: vinegar that is the by-product of making umeboshi plums. Salty and sour, umeboshi vinegar is used as a seasoning in dressings and vegetable dishes.

Wakame: a long, thin sea vegetable used in soups and sometimes in bean dishes. Also used in condiments and pressed salads.

BIBLIOGRAPHY

Aihara, Herman. *Acid and Alkaline.* Oroville, Calif.: George Ohsawa Macrobiotic Foundation, 1986.

Atkins, Robert C. *Dr. Atkins' New Diet Revolution.* London: Vermilion, 1992.

Benedict, Dirk. *Confessions of a Kamikaze Cowboy: A True Story of Discovery, Acting, Health, Illness, Recovery and Life.* Garden City Park, N.Y.: Avery, 1991.

Bumgarner, Marlene Anne. *The New Book of Whole Grains.* New York: St. Martin's Griffin, 1997.

Colbin, Annemarie. *The Book of Whole Meals.* New York: Ballantine, 1983.

———. *Food and Healing.* New York: Ballantine, tenth anniversary edition, 1996.

Dufty, William. *Sugar Blues.* New York: Warner, 1975.

Esko, Edward, ed. *Doctors Look at Macrobiotics.* Tokyo and New York: Japan Publications, 1988.

Faulkner, Dr. Hugh. *Physician Heal Thyself.* Becket, Mass.: One Peaceful World Press, 1992.

Gagne, Steve. *Energetics of Food: Encounters with Your Most Intimate Relationship.* Santa Fe: Spiral Sciences, 1990.

Haas, Elson M., M.D. *Staying Healthy with the Seasons.* Berkeley, Calif.: Celestial Arts, 1981.

Jack, Alex, and Gale Jack. *Amber Waves of Grain: American Macrobiotic Cooking.* Tokyo and New York: Japan Publications, 1992.

Kushi, Aveline, and Wendy Esko. *The Changing Seasons Macrobiotic Cookbook.* Wayne, N.J.: Avery, 1985.

Kushi, Michio. *The Book of Macrobiotics.* Tokyo and New York: Japan Publications, revised edition, 1987.

———. *The Gentle Art of Making Love.* Garden City Park, N.Y.: Avery, 1990.

———. *The Macrobiotic Way.* Garden City Park, N.Y.: Avery, 1985.

———. *Natural Healing through Macrobiotics.* Tokyo and New York: Japan Publications, 1978.

Kushi, Michio, and Aveline Kushi. *Macrobiotic Pregnancy and Care of the Newborn.* Tokyo and New York: Japan Publications, 1983.

Kushi, Michio, with Alex Jack. *The Cancer Prevention Diet.* New York.: St. Martin's Griffin Press, 1993.

Matsumoto, Kosai II. *The Mysterious Japanese Plum*. Santa Barbara, Calif.: Woodbridge Press Publishing Company, 1978.

Ohsawa, George. *Essential Ohsawa: From Food to Health, Happiness to Freedom*. Garden City Park, N.Y.: Avery, 1994.

———. *Macrobiotics: The Way of Healing*. Oroville, Calif.: George Ohsawa Macrobiotic Foundation, 1981.

———. *Philosophy of Oriental Medicine: Key to Your Personal Judging Ability*. Oroville, Calif.: George Ohsawa Macrobiotic Foundation, revised edition, 1991.

———. (as Sakurazawa Nyoiti). *You Are All Sanpaku*. New York: Award Books, 1965.

———. *Zen Macrobiotics*. Los Angeles: The Ohsawa Foundation, 1965.

Ohsawa, Lima. *Macrobiotic Cuisine*. Tokyo and New York: Japan Publications, 1984.

Pirello, Christina. *Cook Your Way to the Life You Want*. New York: HP Books, 1999.

———. *Cooking the Whole Foods Way*. New York: HP Books, 1997.

Pitchford, Paul. *Healing with Whole Foods*. Berkeley, Calif.: North Atlantic Books, revised edition, 1993.

Saltzman, Joanne. *Amazing Grains*. Tiburon, Calif.: HJ Kramer, Inc., 1990.

Stanchich, Lino. *The Power Eating Program: You Are How You Eat*. Coconut Grove, Fla.: Healthy Products Inc., 1989.

Thank God for the Internet. These days, it's incredibly easy to find macrobiotic people and supplies from your home keyboard. That being said, here's some guidance on what you can find.

MACROBIOTIC COUNSELORS

If you are dealing with a serious health condition, you may want to seek the advice of an experienced macrobiotic counselor. There are many counselors out there. But because they have no national governing body, you can't always be sure of what you are getting. Some important questions to ask may be: how long have you been a counselor? Is it your primary profession? Where did you study? Those who make their living as counselors and who have studied with some of the counselors mentioned below may be your best bet for advising you on a serious health issue. Just as important, ask if he or she has worked with any clients with your particular health problem. Get the names of at least three people with whom he or she has worked (with or without your condition) and speak to them directly.

THE RICHEST RESOURCES FOR COUNSELORS

The International Macrobiotic Directory, produced by Robert Mattson. This is a great resource with local addresses and numbers in all states. To order, e-mail him at intermac@earthlink.net or call 510-601-1763. Strengthenhealth.org is Denny Waxman's institute. This faculty consists of very good counselors. The Kushi Institute has counselors.

NAMES OF COUNSELORS WHO HAVE BEEN AROUND A LONG TIME

Michio Kushi (Brookline, Mass.), Marc Van Cauwenberghe (Brookline, Mass.), William Spear (Litchfield, Conn.), Lino Stanchich (Asheville, N.C.), Denny Waxman (Philadelphia, Pa.), David Briscoe (Oroville, Calif.), Joshua Rosenthal (New York), Blake Gould (Morrisville, Vt.), Verne Varona (Los Angeles), Mina Dobic (Los Angeles), Warren Kramer (Boston), Carry Wolf (Becket, Mass.), John Kozinski (Becket, Mass.).

PLACES TO STUDY

The Kushi Institute in western Massachusetts
Strengthening Health Institute in Philadelphia
Institute for Integrative Nutrition in New York City

The Natural Gourmet Cookery School (not "macrobiotic" per se, but very health supportive and delicious food)

WEB SITES TO CHECK OUT

amberwaves.org (Web site to help save organic rice and wheat—good recipes, too)
atasteofhealth.org (healthy vacations organized by Sandy Pukel)
breastcancersurvivors.com (developed by survivor Meg Wolff)
christinacooks.com (Christina Pirello's site)
cybermacro.com (good recipes and resources)
enjoy-life.com (Foundation for the Macrobiotic Way)
gomf.macrobiotic.net (George Ohsawa foundation Web site)
healingcuisine.com (a Web site by chef Meredith McCarty)
integrativenutrition.com (the Institute for Integrative Nutrition)
kushiinstitute.org (the Kushi Institute in Becket, Massachusetts, and its store)
macroamerica.com (Web site by David and Cynthia Briscoe of northern California)
macrobioticcooking.com (a Web site by chef Linda Wernhoff)
macrobiotic.co.uk (the Macrobiotic Association of Great Britain)
macrobiotic.org (Carbondale, Colorado, center for macrobiotics)
macrobioticscanada.ca (a retreat and counseling center in Almonte, Ontario)
macrobioticsnewengland.com (organized by macrobiotic counselor Warren Kramer)
naturalgourmetschool.com (Natural Gourmet School Web site)
Online International Macrobiotic Directory (macrobioticdirectory.com)
rosanna.com (Rosanna's Macrobiotic Kitchen)
strengthenhealth.org (Strengthening Health Institute run by Denny Waxman in Philadelphia)
worldmacro.org (includes newsletter *Non Credo* by Yogen Kushi)

FOOD SOURCES

Diamond Organics (diamondorganics.com or 1-888-ORGANIC)
The Eden Food Company (edenfoods.com or 1-888-441-EDEN)
Goldmine Natural Food Company (goldminenaturalfood.com)
Great Eastern Sun (great-eastern-sun.com or 1-800-334-5809)
The Kushi Institute Store (kushiinstitute.com or 413-645-8744)
Lima Foods Co. (limafood.com)
Maine Coast Sea Vegetables (seaveg.com or 207-565-2907)
The Natural Import Company (1-800-324-1878)
Quality Natural Foods (qualitynaturalfoods.com or 1-888-392-9237)
South River Miso (southrivermiso.com or 413-369-4299)

GREAT COOKBOOK AUTHORS

Christina Pirello, Annemarie Colbin, Aveline Kushi, Meredith McCarty, Kristina Turner, Joanne Saltzman, Marilu Henner, Wendy Esko, Cornelia Aihara, Lima Ohsawa, Boy George, Anya McAteer.

INDEX

Abundance, 160
Acidity, 98, 117, 119
Adrenal glands, 143
Aduki Beans with Squash and Kombu, 213–14
Agar agar, 222
  Strawberry Kanten with Creamy Topping, 139–41
Aggressive behavior, 99
Alcohol, 141–42, 249
Alkalinity, 82
All Hail Hijiki, 222–23
Amaranth and Apricots, 92–93
Amasake, 132
  Mochazake Pie, 233–34
Animal food, 152
Apple-Blueberry Crisp, 237–38
Arame, 222
  Tofu Dumplings, 224–25
Arrogance, 247
Artificial sweeteners, 131
Attraction, 32–35, 271–73
Autumn, 62–63
  menu, 173–74

Baked flour products, 135, 249
Baked Wakame with Onion and Squash, 224
Balanced meals, 161–65

Barley, 76
  Mediterranean Salad, 86–87
Barley malt, 132
Beans, 151, 211–12. See also Tofu
  Aduki, with Squash and Kombu, 213–14
  Black, and Corn Bread Casserole, 219–20
  Black-Eyed Pea Croquettes, 218–19
  Hummus, 216–17
  Mock Tuna (tempeh), 215
  Red Lentil-Walnut Pâté, 212–13
  Scrambled Tofu, 217–18
Bedtime fast, 177
Beverages, 155–56. See also Smoothies
  Carrot-Daikon Drink, 183
  Daikon Drink, 183
  Shiitake Mushroom Tea, 182
Black Bean and Corn Bread Casserole, 219–20
Black-Eyed Pea Croquettes, 218–19
Bladder, 63
Blood pH, 128
Blood sugar imbalances, 107
Body scrub, 176–77
Boiled Salad with Pumpkin-Seed Dressing, 203–205
Brain, 72, 101, 248

Buckwheat, 76
Bulghur wheat, 136

Caffeine, 142–44, 249
Cake, Couscous, 238–39
Calcium, 117, 141
Carbohydrates, 73, 127
Carrot-Daikon Drink, 183
Casein, 119
Centrifugal force, 22–27, 46–47
Centripetal force, 22–27, 46–47
Chakras, 23–24, 251
Change, 19–22
Chaos, 20–21
Cheese, 118
Chemical preservatives, 145–46
Chewing, 80–83
Chicken, 107–108
Chickenless Chicken Salad, Christina's, 109–10
Chips
  Kombu, 188
  Mochi, 187–88
Chocolate Milk Shake, Your New, 121–22
Chocolate Peanut Butter Cups, 133–34
Christina's Chickenless Chicken Salad, 109–10
Clitoris, 263

Coffee, 142
Colorful Harvest Salad, 206–207
Condiments, 155, 239
    Gomashio, 240–41
    Nori, 241
Contraction, 23, 64–66
    attributes created by, *24–25 table*
Cooking plan, 165–68
Corn, 78
    Chowdah, 228
    Pona Lisa, 219–20
Couscous
    Cake, 238–39
    Elegant Orange, 137–38
Cow's milk, 117
Creativity, 252
Crispy Rice Treats, 132–33

Daikon, 112
    Dried, with Dried Tofu, 199–200
    Drink, 183
Dairy food, 114
    benefits from, 118
    problems with, 114–18
    substitutes for, 118–19
       recipes, 119–26
Depression, 128
Desludging, 242–47
Desserts, 153
    Apple-Blueberry Crisp, 237–38
    Couscous Cake, 238–39
    Mochazake Pie, 233–34
    Pears with Ginger Glaze and Pecan
       Cream, 235
    Really Yummy Oat Bars, 236
    Seaweed Nut Crunch, 236–37
    Strawberry Kanten with Creamy
       Topping, 139–41, 233
Diet. *See* Standard Macrobiotic Diet
Dip sauces
    Nabe, 210–11
    Tempura, 198
Discharge, 244
Dreams, pursuing, 253–54
Dried Daikon with Dried Tofu, 199–200
Drugs, recreational, 146
Duality, 18
Dufty, William, 128
Dulse, 222

Eating out, 171–72
Eggs, 107–108
Electrical machinery, 179

Elegant balanced meal, 164–65
Elegant Orange Couscous, 137–38
Emotions, 249–50
Energy
    from meat, 102
    movement in the world, 247–54
    from pursuit of dreams, 253–54
    transformations, 59–64
Erection, 264
Exercise, 180, 250–51
Exercising inner compass
    attraction to similarity, 68
    centers and peripheries of objects, 47
    changes witnessed every day, 66
    eat a cup of brown rice, 26–27
    experiences of attraction, 34–35
    experiences of repulsion, 38
    feelings about change, 22
    nothing is neutral, 48–49
    sensing energies between different
       things, 51
    think about a creative force, 19
    yin and yang in all things, 46
Expansion, 23, 64–66
    attributes created by, *24–25 table*
Expression, 252–53

Farm-raised fish, 112
Fermentation, 118, 141
Fish, 102, 112–14
    Fried Wraps with Asian Coleslaw and
       Rice, 113–14
Flour products, 248
Food. *See also* Recipes; Standard Macro-
       biotic Diet
    additives, 145–46
    beans, 151, 211–20
    for better relationship, 271–73
    beverages, 155–56
    condiments, 239–41
    desserts, 233–39
    extremes, 96–97
       alcohol, 141–42
       caffeinated, 142–44
       chicken and eggs, 107–108
       dairy food, 114–26
       fish, 112–14
       fruit, 139–41
       genetically modified foods,
          144–45
       nightshade vegetables, 141
       red meat, 97–107
       sugar, 126–34

       white-flour products, 134–35
       whole-grain flour, 135–38
    garnishes, 155
    grains, 184–90
    home remedies, 181–83
    occasional, 152–53
       seasonings, 156
    pickles, 155, 231–33
    salt, 153–55
    sea vegetables, 151, 221–25
    soups, 152, 225–31
    vegetables, 149–50, 190–211
    whole grains, 149
    yin and yang of, 25–26, 95–96, *96*
       table
Fried
    Basmati Rice, 91–92
    Fish Wraps with Asian Coleslaw and
       Rice, 113–14
    Noodles, 186–87
Fries, Rutabaga, 194
Fruit, 139–41, 152
    Apple-Blueberry Crisp, 237–38
    juice, 132
    Pears with Ginger Glaze and Pecan
       Cream, 235
    Smoothie, 122
    Strawberry Kanten with Creamy
       Topping, 139–41, 233

Gall bladder, 60
Garnishes, 155
Gay relationships, 262
Genetically modified foods, 144–45
Glossary, 276–79
Glow (Pirello), 178
Glucose, 82, 101
Gomashio, 240–41
Good Morning Oat Porridge, 88
Grains, 184. *See also* Whole-grain flour;
       Whole grains
    Fried Noodles, 186–87
    Hambulghur Helper, 189–90
    Kombu Chips, 188
    Mochi Chips, 187–88
    Mochi Waffles, 188–89
    Steamed Sourdough Bread, 185–86
Gratitude, 180–81
Greens, Steamed, 201

Hambulghur Helper, 189–90
Hato mugi, 78
Healing balanced meal, 163

Health, 247
Hijiki, 222
   All Hail, 222–23
Home remedies, 181–83
Hormones, 101–102
Hot baths, 178
Human milk, 117
Human yin and yang, 23, 25
Hummus, 216–17

Infinite Universe, 16–18, 247, 254
Insulin, 128
Intuition, 131

Kanten, 233
   Strawberry, with Creamy Topping,
      139–41
Kasha and Cabbage, 93–94
Kidneys, 63
Kinpira, 198–99
Kitchen setup, 157–59
Kombu, 222
   Chips, 188
Kushi, Michio, 1, 148

Lactase, 115
Large intestine, 63
Lasagna, 124–26
Late summer, 62
   menu, 173
Leftovers, 168–70
Lifestyle suggestions, 176–83
List of dishes, 165–66
Liver, 60, 252
Love, 273–74
   relationships, 61–64, 251–52
Lungs, 63

Macrobiotics, 1. See also Standard Macro-
      biotic Diet
   and balance, 161–65
   benefits of, 3–6
   diet, 1–2
   five tips for, 274–75
   lifestyle suggestions, 176–83
   Phase One: Grains, 71–94
   Phase Two: Cupboard Conversion,
      95–146
   Phase Three: Going Whole Hog,
      147–83
   resources, 282–84
   terminology, 276–79
   and whole grains, 2–3

Madonna, 21
Maltitol, 131–32
Mango Laasi, Lisa's, 121
Mannitol, 131–32
Maple syrup, 127, 132
Mayonnaise, Tofu, 123
McDonald's, 40–43
Meal planning, 161–65
Meat, 249
   energetic qualities of, 98–102
   guidelines for eaters of, 102
   substitutes for, 103
      recipes, 103–107
   and sugar, 130
Mediterranean Barley Salad, 86–87
Men
   too much yang in, 267
   too much yin in, 264
   yin and yang sides of sexuality, 270–71
Menstruation, 265–66
Menus
   autumn, 173–74
   late summer, 173
   springtime, 174–75
   summer, 175
   winter, 174
Mercury, 112
Microwaves, 179–80
Milk, 117
Millet, 76
   Mashed "Potatoes" with Mushroom
      Gravy, 90–91
Miso, 154
   Basic Soup, 225–26
   Pickles, 232–33
Mochi, 136–37
   Chips, 187–88
   Waffles, 188–89
Mock
   Greek Salad, 208
   Tuna, 215
Molasses, 127
Mood swings, 128
Muscle dysmorphia, 98
Mushroom Barley Soup, 227

Nabe-Style Vegetables, 208–10
National Dairy Council, 118
Natural body products, 178
Natural materials, 178
Nature, 67
Nightshade vegetables, 141
Nishime Vegetables, 193–94

Noncooks, 160–61
Non Credo, 17, 148
Noodles
   in Broth, 230–31
   Fried, 186–87
Nori, 222
   Condiment, 241
Nuts, 153

Oat Bars, Really Yummy, 236
Oat Porridge, Good Morning, 88
Oats, 76–77
Occasional
   foods, 152–53
   seasonings, 156
Ohsawa, George, 4–5, 16–17, 20–21,
      129, 253–54
One-pot balanced meal, 164
Onion Butter, 194–95
Organic food, 156–57
Orgasm, 263, 268
Osteoporosis, 117
Oxytocin, 271

Pancreas, 62, 107, 128
Peanut Butter Cups, Chocolate, 133–34
Pears with Ginger Glaze and Pecan
      Cream, 235
Perfect Brown Rice, 83–84
Pesticides, 156
Pickles, 155
   Miso, 232–33
   Red Radish Umeboshi, 231–32
Pie, Mochazake, 233–34
The pill, 146
Pirello, Christina, 178
Plants, 179
Polyols, 131–32
Prayer for help, 167–68
Pressed salads, 206–208
Pressure-Cooked Brown Rice with
      Chestnuts, 85
Pumpkin-Seed Dressing, 204–205
Purple Passion Stew, 195–96

Quiche, Tofu, 110–12
Quick balanced meal, 164
Quinoa, 77
   Salad, 89–90

Really Yummy Oat Bars, 236
Recipes
   beans, 211–20

Recipes (*cont.*)
  chicken/egg substitutes, 109–12
  condiments, 239–41
  dairy substitutes, 119–26
  desserts, 233–39
  fish, 113–14
  grain products, 184–90
  home remedies, 181–83
  meat substitutes, 103–106
  pickles, 231–33
  sea vegetables, 221–25
  soups, 225–31
  sugar substitutes, 132–34
  vegetables, 190–211
  whole-grain flour, 137–38
  whole grains, 83–94
Recreational drugs, 146
Red Lentil–Walnut Pâté, 212–13
Red meat, 97–102, 249
Red Radish Umeboshi Pickles,
    231–32
Relationships, 251–52
  food for improving, 271–73
  gay, 262
  love, 61–64
  yin and yang of, 258–62
Relaxing balanced meal, 164
Reproductive organs, 63
Repulsion, 35–43
Resources, 282–84
Restaurants, 171–72
Rice, 75–76
  Avocado, and Corn Salad, 87–88
  Crispy Treats, 132–33
  Dream Chocolate Sundae,
      119–20
  Fried Basmati, 91–92
  Perfect Brown, 83–84
  Pressure-Cooked Brown, with
      Chestnuts, 85
Rice fast, 51–57
Rice milk, 119–20
Rice plant, 64
Rice syrup, 132
Roots and Tops, 211
Rutabaga Fries, 194
Rye, 78

Salads
  Boiled, with Pumpkin-Seed Dressing,
      203–205
  Christina's Chickenless Chicken,
      109–10

  Colorful Harvest, 206–207
  Mediterranean Barley, 86–87
  Mock Greek, 208
  Quinoa, 89–90
  Rice, Avocado, and Corn, 87–88
  Teaser Caesar, 205–206
  Tofu "Egg," 110
Saliva, 82
Salt, 153–55
Saturated fat, 263, 267–68
Sautéed Vegetables, 202
Schizophrenia, 129
Scrambled Tofu, 217–18
Sea salt, 154
Seasonal change, 59–64
Sea vegetables, 151
  All Hail Hijiki, 222–23
  Arame Tofu Dumplings,
      224–25
  Baked Wakame with Onion and
      Squash, 224
  benefits of, 221
  types of, 222
Seaweed Nut Crunch, 236–37
Seeds, 153
Seitan, 103
  Stew, 106
Self-centeredness, 100
Sex, 250
Sexual compulsion, 100
Shiitake Mushroom Tea, 182
Shoyu, 154
Simple balanced meal, 164
Sludge, 7–11, 116, 134–35, 143
Small intestine, 99
Smoothies. *See also* Beverages
  Fruit, 122
  Lisa's Mango Laasi, 121
  Your New Chocolate Milk Shake,
      121–22
Soba, 136
Sorbitol, 131–32
Soup, 152
  Basic Miso, 225–26
  Corn Chowdah, 228
  Mushroom Barley, 227
  Noodles in Broth, 230–31
  Split-Pea, 229–30
  Squash, 228–29
Sour Cream, Tofu, 122–23
Sourdough Bread, Steamed,
    185–86
Soybeans, 119

Soy cheese, 118–19
Soy milk, 119
Spelt, 77
Spirals, 22–23
Spiritual pursuits, 254
Spleen, 62
Split-Pea Soup, 229–30
Spring, 59–61
  menu, 174–75
Sprouted-grain bread, 136
Squash Soup, 228–29
Standard Macrobiotic Diet, 1–2, 148.
      See also individual food groups;
      Recipes
  and abundance, 160
  advice for, 156–57
  beans, 151
  beverages, 155–56
  cooking for noncooks, 160–61
  cooking plan, 165–68
  eating out, 171–72
  garnishes, 155
  getting too yang on, 255–58
  kitchen setup, 157–59
  leftovers, 168–70
  meal planning, balance, 161–65
  occasional foods, 152–53
  occasional seasonings, 156
  pickles, 155
  salt, 153–55
  sea vegetables, 151
  soups, 152
  typical macro day, 170–71
  vegetables, 149–50
  whole grains, 149
  and women, 150
  yangizing and yinnizing, 172–75
Starvation, 3, 5
Steamed
  Greens, 201
  Sourdough Bread, 185–86
Stevia, 131
Stew, Purple Passion, 195–96
Stomach, 62
Strawberry Kanten with Creamy
      Topping, 139–41
Strengthening balanced meal, 164
Sugar, 126–27, 248–49
  problems with, 127–31
  substitutes for, 131–32
    macrobiotic, 132
    recipes, 132–34
Sugar Blues (Dufty), 128

Summer, 61–62
  menu, 175
Sweets, 127

Tabbouleh, 138
Tao, 18–19
Tea, Shiitake Mushroom, 182
Teaching others, 181
Teaser Caesar, 205–206
Teeth, 99
Teff, 78
Television, 180
Tempeh, 103
  Burritos, 103–104
  Reuben with Russian Dressing, 105
Tempura, 196–98
Testosterone, 100, 263, 267
Thanksgiving balanced meal, 165
Thinking, 248–49
Thirst, 177–78
Timer, 166–67
Tofu, 103, 108–109
  Arame Dumplings, 224–25
  "Cheese," 120–21
  "Egg" Salad, 110
  Lasagna, 124–26
  Mayonnaise, 123
  Quiche, 110–12
  Scrambled, 217–18
  Sour Cream, 122–23
Tuna, Mock, 215
Twelve Laws of Change, 5
  Law #1, 16–19
  Law #2, 19–22
  Law #3, 22–27
  Law #4, 32–35
  Law #5, 35–43
  Law #6, 44–46
  Law #7, 46–47
  Law #8, 48–49
  Law #9, 49–51
  Law #10, 58
  Law #11, 58–66
  Law #12, 67–68

Udon, 136
Umeboshi plum, 154
Ume-Sho-Kuzu, 181–82

Vegetables, 64, 149–50, 190
  Boiled Salad with Pumpkin-Seed
    Dressing, 203–205
  Colorful Harvest Salad, 206–207
  cooking styles, 192
  downward-growing, 191–92
  Dried Daikon with Dried Tofu,
    199–200
  Kinpira, 198–99
  Mock Greek Salad, 208
  Nabe-Style, 208–10
  nightshade, 141
  Nishime, 193–94
  Onion Butter, 194–95
  Purple Passion Stew, 195–96
  recipes
    lightly cooked, 201–11
    long-cooked, 192–200
  Roots and Tops, 211
  round or ground, 191
  Rutabaga Fries, 194
  Sautéed, 202
  Steamed Greens, 201
  Teaser Caesar, 205–206
  Tempura, 196–98
  upward-growing, 191
Vibrations, 247

Waffles, Mochi, 188–89
Wakame, 222
  Baked, with Onion and Squash,
    224
Walking, 180
Water, 155–56
Wheat, 77
White-flour products, 134–35
White-meat fish, 112
Whole-grain
  bread, 136
  flour, 135–38
Whole grains, 2–3, 64, 71, 149
  barley, 76
  benefits of, 72, 74–75
  boiling instructions, 80 table
  buckwheat, 76
  chewing, 80–83
  combining, 79
  corn, 78

hato mugi, 78
millet, 76
oats, 76–77
pressure-cooking instructions,
  81 table
quinoa, 77
recipes, 83–94
rice, 75–76
rye, 78
soaking, 78–79
spelt, 77
teff, 78
wheat, 77
Whole-wheat
  couscous, 136
  noodles, 136
Winter, 63–64
  menu, 174
Women, 150
  healthy yin in, 269–70
  and menstruation, 265–66
  too much yang in, 263
  too much yin in, 264–65

Xylotol, 131–32

Yin and yang, 13–15
  adjusting cooking to, 172–75
  attraction and repulsion, 49–51
  attraction between, 32–35
  big attracts small, 67–68
  centrifugal and centripetal,
    22–27
  constant change of, 58
  energy transformations between,
    58–66
  excess yang, 255–58
  of food, 25–26, 95–96, 96 table
  infinite production of, 19–22
  of love, 258–74
  nothing is neutral, 48
  as opposites, 18–19
  of physical objects, 46–47
  repulsion between, 35–43
  tendencies of each in all things,
    44–46
You Are All Sanpaku (Ohsawa),
  129